Dance movement therapy: theory and practice

Edited by Helen Payne

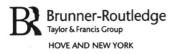
Brunner-Routledge
Taylor & Francis Group

HOVE AND NEW YORK

First published 1992
by Routledge
11 New Fetter Lane, London EC4P 4EE

Simultaneously published in the USA and Canada
by Routledge
29 West 35th Street, New York, NY 10001

Reprinted 1996, 1998 and 1999

Reprinted 2002 and 2004
by Brunner-Routledge
27 Church Road, Hove, East Sussex, BN3 2FA
29 West 35th Street, New York, NY 10001

Brunner-Routledge is an imprint of the Taylor & Francis Group

Typeset in Palatino by Selectmove Ltd
Printed and bound in Great Britain by
TJ International Ltd, Padstow, Cornwall
This publication has been produced with paper manufactured to strict
environmental standards and with pulp derived from sustainable forests.

British Library Cataloguing in Publication Data
Dance movement therapy: theory and practice.
  I. Payne, Helen
  615.85155

Library of Congress Cataloguing in Publication Data
Dance movement therapy: theory and practice / edited by Helen Payne.
  p.cm.
  Includes bibliographical references and index.
  1. Dance therapy.   I. Payne, Helen, 1951-
  RC498.D36   1991
  615.8´5155–dc20

ISBN 0–415–05659–4 (hbk)
ISBN 0–415–05660–8 (pbk)

To my parents, with love

MOVING FROM WITHIN
Lynn Crane

Moved to stillness
    Listening
An inner impulse beckons me to move
Slowly,
I enter that familiar place
    Dance
Immersing myself in movement,   feelings   thoughts
               rhythm,   images,
The essence of my being expressing itself
A movement speaks to me   Discovering
             Dialoguing   Clarifying
Spiralling into the floor where once again stillness calls
I hear the echo of a long lost part of me.
Lying quietly,
Tears flowing
Still waters
Awareness of breath
Rising falling
Rising falling
The dance of life.

Contents

Contributors

Lynn Crane, before moving to live in the UK, studied dance at University of California Los Angeles and continued her postgraduate studies at the Laban course in movement and dance with reference to special education. She was a co-founder of the Association for Dance Movement Therapy in 1982 and worked for ten years in a psychiatric hospital and the community pioneering DMT practice. Lynn is presently devoting her time to her family.

Gayle Liebowitz began to work with psychotic patients twelve years ago on a university placement at a New York City psychiatric hospital. Upon completion of her studies in dance and psychology, she moved to London where she combined her interests by taking an MA at Antioch University and pioneering DMT in London hospitals. At present she is employed by Parkside Health Authority as a Dance Movement Therapist and teaches on the DMT courses at St Albans and at the Laban Centre for Movement and Dance. She is an active member of the Executive Council of the Association for Dance Movement Therapy and a representative on the Standing Committee for Arts Therapies Professions.

Jeannette MacDonald trained at the Royal Ballet, London. She has danced with the Royal Ballet Company, the Stuttgart Ballet, and many other European companies. She created the first NHS dance movement therapy post in this country and, whilst working with DMT, she obtained an Open University BA in psychology. Currently Jeanette is a senior dance movement therapist with Exeter Health Service where her caseload is generic. She lectures extensively and leads numerous DMT workshops for members of the caring professions. She is also a respected dance teacher and as Director of Exeter Dance Centre co-ordinates the work of other dance teachers and teaches ballet to students and professionals.

Bonnie Meekums has been one of the pioneers of dance movement therapy in Britain since 1976. She is employed as a dance movement therapist in the NHS (adult psychiatry). Other practice has included child and adolescent psychiatry and five years with parents and children at risk of abuse. She was also a tutor on the St Albans postgraduate Diploma in DMT (CNAA). Bonnie graduated in physiology and biochemistry with psychology subsidiary and later studied dance, theatre, and writing at Dartington College of Arts. In 1990 she obtained her M.Phil. from the University of Manchester and has published several articles on DMT.

Amelie Noack is a psychologist and psychotherapist working with individuals and groups. She was born in Germany and lived in Berlin, where she studied and completed a degree in architecture, followed by a degree in psychology. During this period of studies, which in Germany takes eleven years, she became more involved in psychotherapy; this against a background of the student movement in Europe. She has trained in different fields of psychotherapy including body and movement therapy and analytical psychology. In connection with her personal experience in movement and dance she has been developing her own approach combining these strands. She is currently living and practising in North London and lectures both in this country and in Europe.

Helen Payne, M.Phil., Adv. Dip. Spec. Ed., Cert. Ed., Laban Cert., began working in 1971 developing her practice pioneering DMT in clinics, hospitals, special schools, and social services. Her specialist PE training was based on Laban's analysis of movement, after which she undertook postgraduate training in special education, dance, counselling, and analytic groupwork. Her research was the first in the UK. As a co-founder of the Association for Dance Movement Therapy, which she chaired for several years, she has given much attention to professional issues in DMT. She designed, initiated, and is currently course leader of the first nationally validated training in DMT at St Albans. Her publications include a book and numerous papers. As well as having a small private practice and consultancy, she is enquiring into DMT training issues for her doctorate. She has been in Jungian analysis for three years and her most recent teacher is her 3-year-old daughter.

Kedzie Penfield came to therapy work from dance. Although she has worked with many client groups in institutions, at present her clients are all high-functioning individuals in the community. Originally from the east coast of the USA, Kedzie has lived and worked in Scotland since 1975 when she came to work as the first dance movement therapist at Dingleton Psychiatric Hospital in the Borders. She teaches Laban Movement Analysis, non-verbal communication, and therapy in many local authorities and training institutions throughout Europe. Her qualifications include a Certificate in Psycho-Motor Therapy and the Certificate of Movement Analysis; she holds the senior registration in the USA for a dance therapist (ADTR) and has also trained in T'ai Chi, massage and Action Profiling.

Pamela Ramsden, BA, MBPS, MAPI, was born in Australia, and her earliest love was dance and movement. She studied psychology at Melbourne University and then came to England. Combining her interests by studying at the Laban Art of Movement Studio, she then worked for ten years alongside Warren Lamb as a management consultant. She is a founding member and vice president of Action Profilers International and is also trained as a Gestalt therapist. A partner in her own consultancy, Decision Development, she is engaged in top executive development, team building, and organization development. She is the author of two books.

Kristina Stanton completed her first degree in psychology at the University of Toronto prior to her MA in religious studies at the University of Kent. She then followed courses in DMT at the Laban Centre and is employed in Kent as a dance movement therapist at a Child and Family Therapy Centre and Integrative Support Project, a private fostering organization for abused children. She continues her studies at the Tavistock Clinic where she receives supervision and is currently writing a book called *An Introduction to DMT in Psychiatry*.

Monika Steiner, originally from Austria, studied for a BA in psychology and history and a postgraduate diploma in dance therapy at Haifa University, Israel. Since coming to England she has completed a psychotherapy training at the Institute of Psychotherapy and Social Studies in London. She has taught on the DMT course at Roehampton Institute. Presently she works in private practice and sessionally as a dance movement therapist in psychiatry and as a tutor on the postgraduate Diploma in Dance Movement Therapy (CNAA) at St Albans.

Susan Stockley trained originally as a dancer, but later abandoned this career to study for an English degree. Although she taught English for several years, her heart was still with the dance. She reconnected with her creative path and studied full time on the SESAME course and at the Laban Centre in drama, movement, and dance for special needs. These courses together with the Feldenkrais method acted as a bridge for her current life interests. She is now a senior lecturer in adult education using movement and dance therapeutically with different groups in the community. She is in training as a humanistic psychotherapist and learning to be a mother.

Paul Tosey, Ph.D., BM.Sc., E.Sc., is a staff tutor in the Human Potential Resource Group, the University of Surrey, and an organizational change consultant. After studying business at undergraduate level he conducted research into organizational change at the University of Bath. His special interest was, and continues to be, connections between psychotherapeutic and organizational models of change, the research also being influenced by new paradigm methodology. Formerly a lecturer at the University of Edinburgh, and trained in co-counselling, group dynamics, and Neuro-Linguistic Programming, until recently he managed an organization development and training unit in Haringey Council. He lives with Helen Payne and their daughter Sarah in Hertfordshire and is currently writing about and developing courses on consultancy and the management of change.

Preface

Dance movement therapy (DMT) is new, as are all the arts therapies (art therapy, music therapy and dramatherapy); however, it has been the last to emerge. It now has, like the other arts therapies, its own validated trainings, supervision of professional practice, and research.

Here I would like to share with you the vision for this book. In my dream journal of 1985 I recorded a dream which was rich in insights on many levels; as a literal dream it has relevance to this book which has now reached fruition. The dream gave me an image of chapters in a book entitled 'Dance Movement Therapy: Theory and Practice'. The concept dealt with 'order out of chaos' (I was writing up my M.Phil. so it was timely!). The chapter headings were, sequentially: DMT in special education; with psychiatric in-patients; in day centres; with children suffering from child abuse; with young people; within a group-analytic perspective; in private practice; with older people; and within a Jungian perspective. It seemed like an ordering of stages of growth from the infant autistic through to the spiritual connection with the universe. It was later that I identified these chapter headings as embodying steps on the pathway towards understanding DMT. The book has therefore stressed the contexts of practice for the most part, rather than solely the population. The individual practitioners have elaborated their methodology within specific settings and client groups and represent current practice within one theoretical orientation.

Acknowledgements

First I must thank the contributors who bravely responded to the challenge of putting into words what is beyond words to a large degree. By definition dance movement therapists are not writers by trade, and it must be acknowledged that to communicate in this medium is difficult. However, their learning has come through and I thank them for their trust in my editorial judgement. It has been a privilege to work with them. My thanks go out to all those who have engaged with me in debate and practice: they have helped me to clarify my work. I include here clients, students, colleagues at work, and especially all those participating in my research over the years.

Finally, thanks go to my daughter, Sarah Rebecca, for indulging me with her patience and also to my partner, Paul Tosey, who has been supportive in this endeavour as in so many before.

Helen Payne

Chapter 1

Introduction

Helen Payne

Dance Movement Therapy (DMT)[1] is a diverse, complex but little-known subject area. This book presents a variety of approaches in settings where the practice of dance movement therapy is appropriate, and individual contributions recognize the varied roots of the subject whilst reflecting the practice which has been pioneered and developed in the UK in recent years. Each contributor has extensive experience in a specific setting but theoretical orientations are different and there are considerable differences in the aims followed and the techniques employed in each setting. By presenting these contributions together it has been my intention to provide the reader with a balanced and clear picture of what makes up dance movement therapy, in the acknowledgement that there is no one style or truth.

WHO IS THE BOOK FOR?

The book has been written for students and other DMT practitioners who may wish to broaden their ideas of what it is possible to experience; to find words to express what they have experienced; and perhaps to say, 'No, that's not what I think or believe, for me it has been different'.

It has also been written for practitioners in the fields of dance and physical education, occupational therapy, physiotherapy, teaching (particularly special education), psychology, arts therapies, and the therapies in general. Finally, it should be of great interest to anyone working in complementary approaches in therapy or medicine, to therapists, nurses, social workers, and all those working in the settings mentioned in the chapter titles. These allied professions have students who do special studies or short courses in DMT and who may later decide to train in the area. This book will give them a theoretical reference to help guide their interest. The 'nuts and bolts' sections under the subheading *Techniques* in each chapter will be particularly valuable to anyone wishing to understand what a dance movement therapist does. Throughout the book specialist terminology has been made accessible to readers from other professions.

HOW IS THE BOOK ORGANIZED?

The book is divided into twelve chapters of a similar length, apart from Chapter 3 which is two chapters in one. Authors were asked to write under common main headings for ease of use. An *Introduction* sets out the historical background to the context of the chapter, the client population where appropriate, and the philosophical orientation and theoretical foundation of the author. Any research which is applicable to DMT, the population, or theme under discussion is referenced at the end of the chapter. Under the second section headed *Techniques*, each author describes the 'tool-kit' which they use in their practice. This may include a particular approach or model, specific strategies, goals for therapy, and so on. The third section, and the focus of each chapter, is the *Case Illustration*. This gives the reader a step-by-step description of the application of DMT in the particular context described. At least one case illustration is given with commentary and evaluation. The focus on what actually happens as a way of highlighting the theoretical points made gives the reader an opportunity to reflect on how DMT is processed and understood by practitioners, the sense we make of our DMT practice. Pseudonyms have been used in these examples. *Conclusions* are drawn at the end of the material.

CO-CREATING THE RHYTHM

There is always a 'right moment' for embarking on any project. There are now two validated training courses in dance movement therapy in the UK and several more in the USA. The year before the formal conception of this book the first postgraduate Diploma in Dance Movement Therapy was validated by the Council of National Academic Awards (CNAA) at Hertfordshire College of Art and Design, St Albans. Innovations such as this, together with the increased recognition of dance movement therapy for registration at M.Phil. and Ph.D. levels in our universities, indicate that the subject is gaining in academic credibility. There is also a professional association (Payne 1983) with over 100 members.

At the time of writing, the professional association is considering criteria for the registration of full practising members. A code of ethics has already been finalized. It is hoped that the association will be in a position to invite practising members to register by 1992. This illustrates the field's growth in status and competence as it begins to establish itself as equal in training and standards of practice with the other arts therapies (art, music, and drama). A career structure in the education and health services is being discussed and salary and conditions of work negotiated in line with other arts therapies.

So, although dance movement therapy has been late to develop in the UK, it is now rapidly reaching the position of becoming a discipline in its own right and requires a body of literature to reflect this. This book is one of the first such contributions. Some of the chapters are from home-grown British practitioners, others are from people who have trained abroad but have developed their practice over a long time in the UK. We are privileged to have contributions from some first-generation practitioners who developed their practice in the early 1970s and 1980s as well as from others who are relatively new to the field. All have practised for between five and twenty years, enabling a rich vein of experience to be tapped. Some are involved with training dance movement therapists. From talking with the contributors during the formative period of the book I think it is fair to say they have found the opportunity to articulate and document their ideas about dance movement therapy a challenge to which they have responded with enthusiasm. Although there is some literature from the Americans in the form of books, a regular journal, and numerous articles, this does not seem to satisfy a UK or European audience. Simply because the US and the UK share a language does not mean that US practice and literature are equipped to develop the quality of work in the UK or that the culture in the US is comparable to the context of UK or European practice. The fact that we both communicate in English is not necessarily a tremendous advantage – it has been observed that the British and the Americans are two races divided by a common language. I believe it is vital that we reflect on DMT practice as it exists now in the UK and share this with students and the wider interested public. By doing so we can give ourselves a greater understanding of the questions arising and those solutions we have arrived at from within the contexts in which we find ourselves working. We need to find opportunities to reflect on our practice and one way of doing this is to write about it.

There are some UK texts about early DMT practice, for example, North (1972), Wethered (1973), or Gardner and Wethered (1986), although there is more evidence of practice in articles, for example, Meier (1979), and book chapters, such as Payne (1988). This book aims to give an account of the stage we are now at in our journey towards an understanding of DMT. It is hoped that the book will motivate further documentation of work and promote further dissemination and understanding of DMT practice.

No one model is stressed in the book. In this way the reader is encouraged to think about the most appropriate model for the client and setting in which they work. For students anticipating placements, beginning practitioners, and experienced therapists changing settings the book provides various approaches; for those already in practice as dance movement therapists it provides a rich source of ideas.

In view of the new courses, growing interest from allied professions, and increasing academic recognition, I think there are reasons to be optimistic about the growth of dance movement therapy in the UK. A book such as this is timely and in rhythm with the steps currently under way.

KEY CONCEPTS

The aims and concepts of dance movement therapy are not widely understood outside the profession. I hope the text here and in further chapters will go some way towards introducing the subject to those who have never heard of DMT and towards providing a greater understanding to others with some interest in the field. People who believe there is more to the body, dance, and movement than is found in the trainings for them, or the recreational and educational pursuits using them, may also find this section helpful.

People often ask 'So what is this dance movement therapy anyway?' At its very simplest, dance movement therapy is the use of creative movement and dance in a therapeutic relationship. Dance movement therapists work on their own or in departments, on hospital wards or as part of multi-disciplinary teams. They work one-to-one or with groups using various approaches and techniques. Conditions differ according to the setting's aims, theoretical views, philosophical beliefs, client groups, staff, and environment.

A recent definition of DMT to which the author contributed and which has been adopted by ADMT and the Standing Committee for Arts Therapies Professions[2] embodies two fundamental principles:

> Dance Movement Therapy is the use of expressive movement and dance as a vehicle through which an individual can engage in the process of personal integration and growth. It is founded on the principle that there is a relationship between motion and emotion and that by exploring a more varied vocabulary of movement people experience the possibility of becoming more securely balanced yet increasingly spontaneous and adaptable. Through movement and dance each person's inner world becomes tangible, individuals share much of their personal symbolism and in dancing together relationships become visible. The dance movement therapist creates a holding environment in which such feelings can be safely expressed, acknowledged and communicated.

There is, however, an uncertainty about the nature of DMT and how it works.

There are some common misconceptions about DMT which need identifying before going any further. These include the following ideas: that DMT is only for those clients with physical difficulties such as co-ordination problems; that only people with a natural talent for rhythm or movement should attend DMT; and that only those inexperienced in creative expression need be referred for DMT. There may be clients with all these characteristics in DMT sessions but the referral criteria are not normally on these bases.

For example, working with a trained dancer in DMT will require a very different approach from working with someone who has had no dance training at all. The need to abandon technique in favour of spontaneity is sometimes difficult for dancers and can have the effect of de-skilling, when it is no longer possible to hide behind the body's training.

Another common misunderstanding is that dance movement therapists are simply teachers who work with patients or clients in hospitals or special schools. They may be qualified teachers also but they are trained in other aspects such as self-awareness and skills concerned with reflection on actions within the therapeutic process, for example, transference and counter-transference issues. The relationship between teaching and therapy is addressed more fully in *Chapter 3*.

Linked to this is the idea that in DMT dance artists give others the opportunities to dance and perform, the 'art for all' idea, particularly appropriate in hospitals, prisons, special schools, and so on. The dance movement therapist may have had a dance training and be experienced as a dance performer but they will also have taken further trainings in DMT and have aims and objectives which rarely include working with clients towards a dance performance in the public arena.

Neither is DMT another form of occupational therapy (O.T.), although it is true that some early pioneers were trained in this field and others first introduced the work within O.T. departments. However, these people had further training in, for example, Laban Movement Analysis plus experience of personal therapy and psychotherapy qualifications. Confusion may have arisen because in health settings DMT has usually come under O.T. for the purposes of administration. Special arts therapies departments are now being set up in many hospitals, as separate administrative units, as the acceptance of this work grows and numbers employed increase.

Finally, DMT is at times confused with physiotherapy. The fact that both use the body is probably the reason for this. Although DMT does incorporate movement/dance exercises, perhaps in a warm-up, the focus is not on the execution of these as it is in physiotherapy. Both professions emphasize the goal of increasing movement range, albeit for different reasons, and this can be seen as a similarity, but it is the unconscious and symbolic aspects of communication which are the focus in DMT.

There is shared understanding between dance movement therapists and some occupational therapists, physiotherapists, and psychologists in relation to the connection between exercise and stress release. The historical context of Western and non-Western dance eustress/stress has been addressed by Hanna (1988) from an anthropological perspective. In an important research study Leste and Rust (1984) found anxiety levels decreased in the dance experimental group in comparison to music therapy and physical education control groups. The cathartic nature of dance, with its concomitant of insight, releases the tension built up by stress, bringing relief. The Greeks equated dance with catharsis. Dance movement (like other movement forms) is a pleasurable expenditure of energy, different from everyday movement, which offers relaxation and sublimation. It can sometimes lead to altered states of consciousness as in, for example, the spinning dance of the Whirling Dervishes. There is a feeling of well-being induced after dancing which suggests that it improves affective states. This is empirically recognized to be the case in most other forms of exercise. Involvement in dance provides for distraction from stressful situations and anxious thoughts. The endorphins produced by the brain and pituitary gland when the body is engaged in physical activity can reduce the perception of pain, acting as a tranquillizer. Vigorous activity and the resulting fatigue can lead to an abatement of rage. Other research (Morgan 1985) suggests that tension reduction after exercise lasts longer than that after meditation or distraction interventions. There is a suggestion that dance increases the levels of the chemical norepinephrine which are reduced in stress-induced depression. So there are valid physiological reasons for the place of dance – exercise in therapy, emphasizing the unique contribution DMT has to make in, for example, the treatment of stress and psychosomatic disorders.

Despite this obvious connection with physical fitness and health, DMT is much more aligned with psychotherapy. In the UK, group-analytic theory has influenced group practice, as have psychoanalytic methods such as free association in movement. This is because the roots of the movement lie in Laban's creative dance form, modern educational dance as it was termed in education (Laban 1975), which developed in the 1940s when some of the first work was begun using the approach with psychiatric patients. However, spontaneous expression is not the therapy in and of itself. It is the transformation of the individual through the medium which becomes the focus in the therapeutic relationship. In UK practice it is not normally considered appropriate for the therapist to interpret the client's movement. This is more widely practised in the US where diagnosis from assessment of movement characteristics is more common also. Despite North's (1972) research involving personality assessment through movement, this approach has not been as popular with UK practitioners, although several have had rigorous training in the methods. It is often easy to observe a disturbed person's emotional condition reflected in their movement and posture, but this is different from saying there are pathologies for which certain movement characteristics are the indicators. However, much of the US literature, such as Dulicai (1977), and Davis (1970), can be used to support the notion that movement assessment is a valid tool for use with people with a variety of difficulties in functioning.

Partly because of necessity, but perhaps also through choice, therapists in the UK work mainly with groups (working with individuals is a very different skill). Therefore the use of movement observation during sessions is necessarily limited and movement profiles are less likely to be as detailed as when applied to an individual. The idea inherent in this practice of non-interpretation of movement patterns comes from the influences of Gestalt therapy and humanistic psychology where it is the client, for whom the meaning has relevance in the personal situation, who, together with the therapist, gives meaning to the work. That is not to say that during reflection on sessions the therapist does not speculate and connect aspects of the client's known life-history and current life-events with movement, verbal, and interactive behaviour. Any movement observations the therapist makes in the session may stimulate suggestions in the session itself and affect the adjustment in objectives or any planning of the following session. The safety of the session and the trust the client establishes with the therapist lead to an openness within which the client can explore their definition of self. DMT is concerned with the evidence that for certain populations of clients, with similar symptoms, some movement characteristics do seem to recur which enable a rough plan to be designed around selecting approach, methods, and techniques thought to be most appropriate. But this is different from the assumption that these movement patterns are reflective of the particular symptoms in general. For example, a depressed patient may walk with a downward focus and a slow gait with inward flow and she may communicate her hopelessness in a movement pattern similar to that of another person (see *Chapter 8, by Kedzie Penfield*). The movement patterns and qualities may be similar, but because a person walks in that manner it does not necessarily imply that the person is therefore depressed. Context is all important here: without looking at the surrounding conditions and talking to the client this method of diagnosis becomes simplistic.

Chapter 11, by Pamela Ramsden, enlarges on the idea of movement assessment in the context of self-development. One of the tools used widely in DMT, Laban Movement Analysis, has been sophisticatedly refined and is used in the context of management development, training, and team building. This makes for an interesting contrast between an aspect of DMT used for the development of professional managers and DMT with those in hospitals, social service settings, and special education. The movement analysis is used with managers and teams in the form of the Action Profile system. Laban's system was developed by Lamb and Watson (1979) and Pamela Ramsden's chapter further refines this work, particularly in relation to motivation and decision-making, which would be of special interest to managers in the caring professions. She has discussed with others in earlier writings (Davis *et al.* 1981) how such movement profiles may be used in DMT assessment. However, although there may be inter-observer reliability about what is seen, it may not be accompanied by agreement on how to interpret it. The Action Profile system represents a social tendency and could be a possible development area for the application of DMT.

Another key concept is that of transference, which occurs when the client transfers strong, often infantile feelings onto the therapist. This concept is crucial to any psychotherapeutic relationship and is important in helping early experiences, which often relate to current situations, to emerge. Even though transference is acknowledged in DMT it is the movement which is the main tool of the therapy process, whereas in classical psychoanalysis it is the transference. *Chapter 3, by Helen Payne,* and *Chapter 5, by Gayle Liebowitz,* discuss this aspect in their case illustrations in more depth. *Gayle Liebowitz,* in particular, talks about the concept of delusional body transference where the therapist's body becomes the reflection of the client's mother's body. Field (1989) describes how the spontaneous arousal of physical feelings in the therapist can be embodied as counter-transference, for example, sexual arousal, sleepiness, or trembling. It is crucial for DMT to address these issues in the effort to differentiate the patient's contribution from the therapist's. By considering unconscious bodily reactions we may grasp a further 'knowing' in the therapeutic encounter. The therapist's body can act as a barometer enabling recognition and understanding of the patient's experience.

Current practice as we now know it has its primary source in the dances of early societies which are still used to bring about healing of mind, body, and spirit. *Amelie Noack, in Chapter 9,* gives an interesting synopsis of the mythological roots of dance. Dance has been used to reflect and transcend trends in society and has traditionally been used for personal expression individually and in groups. The validity of this practice has long been recognized. In DMT its distinct purpose is to engage the person spontaneously in the process of moving, not to produce a dance or to create movements to form a performance. Creativity is not the main focus although it has been acknowledged that the creative process in itself can also be therapeutic. Aesthetic considerations are not of importance in DMT. When DMT is engaged in it is acknowledged that a therapy contract is entered into. There are normally clear aims and objectives related to overall treatment aims. The presence of the therapist is vital to the process and there are different purposes from dance or movement forms used for recreation, education, or as a performance art. The person and the process are the crucial elements in therapy and in DMT these elements take priority; together with the use of movement as the form of non-verbal communication, they act as agents for therapeutic change. These elements of the person, process, and non-verbal communication are the common ground shared by the arts therapies. The movement activity in DMT is a concrete medium through which conscious and unconscious expression can become motivated. The most usual aim of therapy is dealing with problems of relationship. By the intentional use of relationship therapy can aim to bring about durable, positive change with someone whose potential in relating has become problematic. Unformed feelings may become clarified as a result of the process. In DMT it is recognized that feelings derived from the unconscious reach expression in movement (or its creative form, dance) rather than words. This includes images emerging from the movement described by *Kristina Stanton in Chapter 6*, where she stresses that the group's use of imagery and metaphor is derived from the movement interaction thus acting as a vehicle for transformation. Therapy then is not seen to be a consequence of simply engaging in moving creatively, hence it is different from creative dance. Until a decade ago dance in education was seen as creative dance in the main, separate from dance in theatre, where technique and performance were more important than process. However, now dance in education has begun to stress technical aspects, aesthetics, and performance, and dance theatre has recently been engaging with process work.

I would now like to draw your attention to the poem 'Moving From Within' by *Lynn Crane* which prefaces this book. This expresses something central to the book. It reminds me of what Jung (1961) said in *Memories, Dreams, Reflections* with reference to the self: 'The self is the principle and archetype of orientation and meaning. Therein lies its healing function' (Jung 1961: 224). The essence of DMT has a deep connection with finding a way to facilitate the emergence of opposites, such as movement and stillness contained within the totality of the self.

Moving is fundamental to life, and the capacity for it is universal. The rhythmic beat of the solar system is reflected in our world, in its relationship to our sun and moon, the seasons, night and day, the beating of our hearts, the flow of our breath, the cycle of life and death. In DMT rhythm can provide a holding factor for some clients where moving in silence is too threatening, and can unite a group by communicating through synchronous movement activity. The ability to communicate is a primary human characteristic. If speech is one means of communication, movement is another, more direct form. The pre-verbal symbols which emerge can clarify a thought or feeling more easily for many clients (see *Kedzie Penfield, Chapter 8*). For those with a learning difficulty or speech impairment, movement can symbolize their conflicts and give a new meaning to their inner world. *Jeannette MacDonald, in Chapter 10,* enlarges on this point. That is not to say speech is not used in DMT. Both *Kristina Stanton* and *Gayle Liebowitz* illustrate the role verbalization can have in discussion of movement interactions afterwards with the therapist. This enables a cognitive insight, previously hidden, to become clear. There may be a cathartic reaction in some clients, where they become absorbed because of the physical and emotional involvement of the work. Powerful emotions may be expressed in this way. It is vital that the experience is resolved and integrated, however. The actual process of moving can engender strong feelings, as shown in Reich's important work using breathing (Reich 1945) and later work popularized by Lowen (1976) in bioenergetics. Totton and Edmonson (1988) give an up-to-date account of Reich's pioneering insights and techniques. His contribution to DMT cannot be underestimated. This includes, for example, concepts such as body armouring and the idea that areas of the body 'hold' memories of early experiences such as birth trauma. The body memory can begin to recall earlier pleasant or unpleasant experiences through movement sparking off the muscle memory. There is an inherent safety in the DMT approach because movement is there and then gone in a split second, like play in a sense; it is almost impossible to recapture a spontaneous movement exactly a second time. In this way some clients find it more accessible.

Words are placed at the top of society's ladder of valuable forms of communication – one reason why this book has been written. There is less importance attached to the arts in general, and the ambiguity of dance in particular, unless purely representational, often leaves people unsure of what exactly it is trying to say. Dance attracts stereotypes, and the way a client sees dance or movement or therapy will colour their attitude to the process and their subsequent benefit from it.

Jungian thought in DMT has had little attention until recently. Jungians define creativity as arising from the unconscious depths, giving form to feelings, thoughts, and beliefs. *Amelie Noack, in Chapter 9,* gives a fascinating insight into how the symbol of the tree provides the form for an understanding of movement expression within the therapeutic context. *Helen Payne (Chapter 3)* suggests that for some clients the group-analytic dance approach is more appropriate, encouraging free association of movement to reflect the inner processes.

In *Chapter 2 Bonnie Meekums* uses what could be termed a behavioural approach to DMT by the use of reinforcement techniques in the form of praise from the therapist with 'at risk' children and their mothers. A strictly behaviourist approach would use DMT to modify clients' behaviour towards cultural and social norms. The emphasis here is on the acquisition of skills as in assertiveness training, such as saying 'no' with an upright posture and a forward gaze. I am not sure whether behavioural approaches in general can be therapy in the sense that they aim to teach techniques, but they have been found helpful with phobias and some aspects of delinquent behaviour or learning/communication difficulties.

Monika Steiner, in Chapter 7, presents an interesting model which uses all three approaches: Social learning (behavioural), existential-holistic, and psychodynamic. Her contribution describes the role of DMT in a therapeutic community with a psychiatric group. It explores how the hostel in the community can become a bridge for psychiatry. Issues such as prevention and rehabilitation are addressed as is the healing power of communal dance when engaged with in the framework of group processes.

HISTORICAL DEVELOPMENT

It was in the 1940s that dance first began to be used in psychiatry and then later was evolved in special education, family work, work with older people, and with people with learning disabilities. The unique British system of health, education, and social services has been fundamental to the development of ideas and attitudes towards therapy in general and DMT in particular. Although there was some isolated practice in psychiatric hospitals, it was not until the mid 1970s that groups came into being to offer informal trainings and support networks. At this time also, the SESAME course in movement and drama in therapy and the Laban Centre's one-year full-time course on dance in special education went some way towards establishing a specialism, where movement observation and dance therapy were components (see Appendix for map of the development and flow of DMT training).

In the late 1970s and early 1980s a small group of practitioners, some of whom had completed the Laban Centre course, began to meet on an informal basis to offer each other supervision and support. From 1976 *Kedzie Penfield*, in particular, helped an emergence of understanding in our work and supported us through supervision, skills workshops, and personal process. Guest teachers from America were invited to lead open workshops and intensive events, particularly Dr Joanna Harris who gave emotional strength to the idea of developing a professional association (Harris 1980). It was out of this support group that, in

London in 1982, a more formal organization emerged, the Association for Dance Movement Therapy (ADMT) (Payne 1983). Three members of the support group were its founders: Lynn Crane, Catalina Garvie, and the author, although others also invested time and energy.

In 1985 an American training was imported to the Laban Centre and by 1987 a non-validated college training had been set up at Froebel College, Roehampton Institute, again taught by a leading American practitioner. As well as this American input, pioneers of UK practice during the 1970s and 1980s developed their own style of working influenced by, for example, Laban's creative dance, classical and modern dance, Gestalt therapy, group analysis, Reichian therapy, and object relations and Jungian theories. Despite these beginnings, DMT in the UK was still in the position of having no validated and recognized training, the only arts therapy still without a university or CNAA postgraduate diploma-level course as an initial training programme. However, it was the team at Hertfordshire College of Art and Design, St Albans, led by the author who took the initiative and successfully developed such a course. With over twenty years' experience in arts therapies training they were able to establish a course consistent with the other postgraduate training courses in the UK in art therapy, dramatherapy, and music therapy. The postgraduate Diploma in Dance Movement Therapy was awarded CNAA validation in 1988. The Laban Centre for Movement and Dance followed with a similar development for DMT training in 1989, with American staffing. The two courses, although both now standardized by CNAA validation, offer a slightly different emphasis and approach, particularly since their historical roots are in UK and US practice respectively. For example, the St Albans course stresses that participation in a DMT group experience is essential to the learning process as part of the programme and, in addition, strongly recommends that students engage in individual personal therapy.

UK practitioners have struggled to evolve a profession, training, and practice culturally acceptable to our work settings and society here. They have been greatly helped by the hard work of colleagues in the other three arts therapies who had professional associations, established and recognized trainings, and NHS recognition. More recently art therapy has become recognized in social services and dramatherapy is in similar negotiations. There is a joint arts therapies committee working towards recognition in the education service (see Appendix for the address). In addition, a more recent development is a combined move towards forming a section for arts therapies in the UK Standing Conference for Psychotherapy.

In America the story is different. Dance therapy initiatives began in the 1960s when the professional body, the American Dance Therapy Association (ADTA), under the leadership of Marian Chace, was formed in 1966. The Association has over 1,500 members and two levels of registration, the most senior having over 350 members. Influences in the early days were from modern dance trainings rather than the Laban approach. Courses have been under way for over a decade and at least seven courses are at MA level. Other courses are undergraduate or creative arts therapies based.

There are currently no state-funded or nationally validated post-graduate trainings in DMT in other parts of Europe, although private centres do exist. There are networks of practitioners rather than established professional associations. Holland has an undergraduate course and postgraduate trainings in psychomotor therapy and post-doctoral training in integrative movement therapy. There is interest in Germany, France, and Sweden, and in Italy an independent American course, Art Therapy Italiana, has a DMT component (see Appendix for addresses).

In summary, there has been an energetic development of DMT in the UK emerging from many contributions in recent years. This cannot be seen as a simple linear development but, like the process of DMT itself, as an interactive one, with many influences permeating it along the way. DMT is such a new field that it is constantly defining itself. The chapters in this book reflect this process. The orientations of contributors are mirrored in the stresses they place on application, some giving guidelines for practice, others clarifying theoretical concepts, and yet others presenting more case illustrations. In giving an overview of some approaches to dance in remedial and therapeutic fields, some chapters emphasize the process more than others but no one approach can be said to be the only way – all are truths.

WHAT DOES A DANCE MOVEMENT THERAPIST DO?

A range of client populations are referred for DMT. Some have no hope of recovery, such as the severely mentally handicapped, learning disabled, or physically handicapped. Others, such as delinquent or emotionally disturbed children/adolescents, psychiatric patients, families, and so on, are in appropriate rehabilitation or treatment programmes, whilst still others can be engaged in growth with a less curative emphasis such as older people, long-term institutionalized normal neurotics like you and me, and so on. Whereas DMT was used with the chronic long-term populations on back wards of the large hospitals, now, with the move into the community, these institutions are emptying and DMT too is moving out into day centres, hostels, and other community settings. *Monika Steiner* gives an overview of what the implications of this recent government initiative are for her DMT practice.

A more specialized form of DMT is working with the family. Move ment is used as a means of communication and to understand how mother and child relate as a dyad, for example. *Bonnie Meekums* describes her approach to DMT when working with child and mother, together with other dyads.

There is often confusion between teaching dance and DMT. *Helen Payne, in Chapter 3*, describes the tensions of working in a special school setting as a dance movement therapist and *Susan Stockley, in Chapter 4*, presents her approach to DMT with older people which took place under the auspices of adult education. She particularly examines the issue of ageism and the taboo of death. DMT can be of great help in transcending the difficulties surrounding those who are coming to the end of their life and facing the imminence of death. Those individuals ageing in cultures with few expectations and roles for older people can become depressed from a sense of losing their ability to adapt to the environment. The accompanying limited movement capability and co-ordination, and increase in bodily ailments, contribute to low self-esteem. Ageing too can be viewed in terms of stress.

Generally DMT sessions have an introductory warm-up time followed by a period of initiation into the process of moving individually or as a group in a spontaneous and deeper way. Finally there is a warm-down stage which integrates and focuses participants on the closure of the session. The therapist may explain at the outset the aim of the session and how this might be achieved. The session might be directed by concentrating on a specific theme selected by the client or in conjunction with the therapist, or material emerging in previous sessions. It may be non-directed, where the group move, or not, concluding with verbal processing. Groupwork naturally engenders powerful dynamics. Normally the theme provides a focus through which individuals relate their personal meaning. There may be a sense of competition, regression, or inhibition when working with groups in DMT. Sometimes clients remember childhood failures in movement or dance at school, and resistance may be expressed in statements like 'This is stupid' or 'I can't move/dance' or 'You can't make me into a dancer'. How the work is communicated is vital, as are facilitator styles when working in a group. Many groupwork techniques addressing these and other practical issues are described in depth in Payne (1990).

Although much of the time the therapist moves with the client and acts as a participant as well as an observer, the dance movement therapist must also learn how to refrain from interfering with the movement material presented by the client. The need to interpret is often the therapist's need to make the comment. By waiting or first asking the client to attempt an explanation of the content and meaning of the movement statement the therapist can help a further exploration and understanding through a shared dialogue and then possible interpretation by the therapist. It is dangerous to make premature interpretations; it is often the inexperienced or unskilled therapist who does this. Whilst on the subject of interpretation, *Paul Tosey*, who is a non-practitioner, takes a look, in the final chapter, at the other chapters and gives meaning to what he has absorbed. From his perspective a reflection is presented on those themes and issues which have arisen in the practitioners' sections of the book. There is a metaphor used about the process of a snake shedding its skin. Contradictions, similarities, and theoretical concepts are identified as patterns which give a frame of reference to the reader. This chapter aims to capture the essence of DMT at the moment and gives the reader insight into what and how dance movement therapists communicate to others, outside the profession, what we actually do and understand about this 'doing'.

Finally, it must be stressed that to be a successful dance movement therapist it is essential to engage in regular supervision with an experienced practitioner outside the setting.

THE FUTURE

More research is vitally needed in the areas of processes, practices, assessment, and movement observation in DMT theory and practice, particularly in those settings where empirically DMT has been found to be valuable. Far more research has taken place in the US, particularly in the area of clinical results where there has been an emphasis on the traditional approaches to research which easily dovetail with areas such as efficacy and diagnosis. Related studies into areas such as psychotherapy, body image, and non-verbal communication have come from psychological fields. There is also anthropological research of relevance, for example Spencer (1985) and Hanna (1990), and a wealth of research studies in aspects of exercise physiology and stress. Published research on DMT to date in the UK is small, but in contrast to the US has focused on the in therapy processes and evaluative methodologies from the emerging approaches to enquiry developing in the human sciences (Reason and Rowan 1981; Reason 1988; Lincoln and Guba 1985). One of the major criticisms of research using the experimental approach is that it fails to take account of the interactive nature of human beings; if DMT is to convince others of its value it needs to explore such post-positivist approaches to research; the more traditional ones have failed to 'prove' its effectiveness. A beginning has been made in the few UK studies to date. The use of quantitative methods alone does not seem to have been appropriate. I have argued the reasons for this elsewhere (Payne 1992). Given these difficulties, one way of researching the processes involved in

DMT is to ask the clients (Payne 1988). An understanding of the clients' perceptions has been found to provide useful information about how DMT operates with a particular client group, setting, and therapist.

Finally, the future of DMT must lie in the establishment of its recognition by the NHS, education, and social services. A union affiliation which covers these three settings is imperative if DMT is to have the same conditions of service as other arts therapies. It is still a struggle establishing DMT as a valid, respected discipline in the UK. We are currently exploring, for example, state recognition with the Council of Professions Supplementary to Medicine. In the future it will be important to align with our fellow Europeans towards common goals and visions. There has been much achieved but there is still a long way to go. The aim must be to establish DMT in every treatment programme, available to all those in need of care and who have special needs, whether for curative or maintenance goals. To achieve this the profession needs to adopt a collaborative approach and I hope that this book will go part way towards this end.

NOTES

1 In the USA, Dance/Movement Therapy, Dance Therapy, Dance-Movement Therapy, and Movement Therapy are used interchangeably. In the UK Dance Movement Therapy (DMT) is the term in normal usage.
2 The Standing Committee for the Arts Therapies Professions has produced a leaflet for employers which gives an understanding of the nature of *Artists and Arts Therapists: Their Differing Roles, in Hospitals, Clinics, Special Schools, and the Community*; it is available from Stella Mottam, Hertfordshire College of Art and Design, 7 Hatfield Road, St Albans, Herts, England.

REFERENCES

Davis, M. (1970) 'Movement characteristics of hospitalized psychiatric patients', in M. N. Costonis (ed.) *Therapy in Motion*, Chicago: University of Illinois Press, pp. 89–110.
Davis, M., Dulicai, D., Fried, J., Loman, S., and Ramsden, P. (1981) 'Laban-influenced movement profiles: a critical discussion on their reliability, validity and value to dance therapy', *Conference Proceedings, 16th ADTA Annual Conference: Research as a Creative Process*, Madison, Wisconsin.
Dell, C. (1970) *A Primer for Movement Observation*, New York: Dance Notation Bureau Press.
Dubovski, J. (ed.) (1990) 'Arts therapies education – our European future', *Conference Proceedings*, Hertfordshire College of Art and Design, 7 Hatfield Road, St Albans, Herts.
Dulicai, D. (1977) 'Non-verbal assessment of family systems: a preliminary study', *Art Psychotherapy* 4: 55–68.
Field, N. (1989) 'Listening with the body: an exploration in the

counter-transference', *British Journal of Psychotherapy* 5(4): 512–22.

Gardner, C. and Wethered, A. (1986) 'The therapeutic value of movement and dance', in L. Burr (ed.) *Therapy through Movement*, Nottingham: Nottingham Rehabilitation Press.

Hanna, J. (1988) *Dance and Stress*, New York: AMS Press.

——(1990) 'Anthropological perspectives for dance movement therapy', *American Journal of Dance Therapy* 12(2): 115–26.

Harris, J. G. (1980) 'Slowly but surely', *Inscape* 4: 1, British Association of Art Therapists.

Jung, C. G. (1961) *Memories, Dreams, Reflections*, London: Collins and Routledge & Kegan Paul.

Laban, R (1975) *Modern Educational Dance*, third edition, London: Macdonald & Evans.

Lamb, W. and Watson, E. (1979) *Body Code: The Meaning in Movement*, London: Routledge & Kegan Paul.

Leste, A. and Rust, J. (1984) 'Effects of dance on anxiety', *Journal of Perceptual Motor Skills* 58: 767–72.

Lincoln, I. and Guba, E. (1985) *Naturalistic Inquiry*, London: Sage.

Lowen, A. (1976) *Bioenergetics*, London: Coventure.

Meier, W. (1979) 'Meeting special needs through movement and dance drama', *Therapeutic Education* 7(1): 27–33.

Morgan, W. P. (1985) 'Affective beneficence of vigorous physical activity', *Medicine and Science in Sports and Exercise* 17(1): 94–100.

North, M. (1972) *Personality Assessment through Movement*, London: Macdonald & Evans.

Payne, H. L. (1983) 'The development of the Association for Dance Movement Therapy', *New Dance* Winter: 27.

——(1988) 'The use of DMT with troubled youth', in C. Schaefer (ed.) *Innovative Interventions in Child and Adolescent Therapy*, London/New York: Wiley.

——(1990) *Creative Dance and Movement in Groupwork*, Oxon: Winslow.

——(1992) 'The practitioner as researcher: research as a learning process', in H. Payne (ed). *One River, Many Currents*, London: Jessica Kingsley.

Reason, P. (ed.) (1988) *Human Inquiry in Action*, London: Sage.

Reason, P. and Rowan, J. (eds) (1981) *Human Inquiry: A Sourcebook of New Paradigm Research*, Chichester: Wiley.

Reich, W. (1945) *Character Analysis*, New York: Simon & Schuster.

Spencer, P. (ed.) (1985) *Society and the Dance*, Cambridge: Cambridge University Press.

Totton, N. and Edmonson, E. (1988) *Reichian Growth Work*, Bridport, Dorset: Prism Press.

Wethered, A. (1973) *Drama and Movement in Therapy*, London: Macdonald & Evans.

Chapter 2

The love bugs

Dance movement therapy in a Family Service Unit

Bonnie Meekums

INTRODUCTION

This chapter describes a twenty-session dance movement therapy group for four mothers and their four toddlers, the group having been named 'The Love Bugs' by the mothers. The group took place between January and July 1987 at Leeds Family Service Unit (LFSU), all of the children being considered by a social worker to be at risk of abuse prior to DMT. The work formed part of a research project (Meekums 1990), whose pilot study has been previously reported (Meekums 1988). In the absence of other appropriately experienced practitioners in Yorkshire, both the role of dance movement therapist and that of researcher were taken by the author.

The literature on dance movement therapy with mothers and young children is sparse, though there are some descriptive or case study reports of similar work in the USA (Kestenberg and Buelte 1977; Murphy 1979; Ostrov 1981; Bell 1984), and there have been two small studies of such work in England (Graham 1984; Meekums 1988).

There is, however, considerable information on the nature of functional and dysfunctional mother–child interaction. Winnicott's (1965) writings on what he calls the 'holding environment'[1] are of particular relevance to this study. Winnicott suggests that the 'holding environment' is initially 'a three-dimensional or space relationship with time gradually added' (Winnicott 1960: 44). The child's ability to progress towards maturity, according to Winnicott, depends at least in part on the mother's[2] ability to provide a secure holding environment during infancy.

Kestenberg and Buelte (1977) emphasize the importance of adaptive physical holding of the infant by the mother, and vice versa, for later self-reliance. Dulicai's (1977) research suggests that functional families are more likely to display moulding, that is, fitting into or around each other's body shapes, and less likely to exhibit static body attitudes, than are dysfunctional families. Whilst Dulicai used a small sample, her results have been confirmed by others trained by her, including one study concerning adoptive families (Webster 1987). Silberstein (1984) suggests that, for the older child, the tendency towards moulding is replaced to some extent by the mother's frequent glances towards her toddler.

The presence of interactional synchrony[3] as an indicator of empathy has long been assumed (Condon 1968), and Kestenberg (1975) suggests that synchronization of rhythms is necessary for the 'attunement' commonly experienced by mother and infant. A study by Fraenkel (1983), however, suggests that in adult interactions perceived as empathic by the participants, echoing rather than synchrony is an indicator, particularly once interaction is established, whilst synchrony is more prevalent in the first ten minutes. Echoing is perhaps more likely within the framework of a conversation, in which verbalizations do not occur synchronously but in a process of 'give and take'. It is possible that this process is built through the mother's early responses to the infant; both Ostrov (1981) and Schaffer (1977) emphasize the need for the mother to follow the focus of the child, rather than lead. Schaffer (1977) writes of the 'pseudo-dialogue', during which the mother responds to her infant as if they were holding a conversation, and in this way, he claims, the infant learns reciprocity.

TECHNIQUES

During the DMT programme, the following interventions were used:

1 Polaroid photographs of each dyad were taken at the start and near to the end of the group, and each pair glued these onto an individual file in which their interaction was recorded week by week. The purpose of this process was to provide a visual reflection of the pair as a unit, and to encourage each mother to identify with the file, in which progress would be charted by the dance movement therapist.
2 Positive comments were made by the therapist concerning inter-actions to be encouraged, for example, 'that looks like a nice cuddle'.
3 Help was given in changing maladaptive behaviour, for example by suggesting the mother squat and hold the child's hands gently, making eye contact as she explained an instruction.
4 Early in the group, structured activities which encouraged mother-child interaction were used, whilst the group developed in con-fidence. An example of such a structure is 'blankets', in which each child takes a turn to be rocked by the whole group as she or he lies in the centre of a duvet or blanket. The mother is positioned for easy eye contact, and the whole group is encouraged to use a slow, smooth, and gentle rocking motion. The trajectory of the

child's body is an arc, and their body moulds to a foetal position. This activity was found to be useful in establishing rhythmic synchrony and indulging, nurturing movement qualities (Laban 1960; Ostrov 1981), without the need for close physical contact. To force physical contact between mothers and children who are not 'bonded' can be counterproductive, particularly early in therapy.

5 Circles and songs were used throughout the DMT programme as a way of marking the beginning and end of a session, or part of a session.

6 Some structures were used both diagnostically and therapeutically, to assess and develop the mother's ability to protect the child. These included the game, 'What's the time, Mr Wolf?', in which the dance movement therapist pretended to be a wolf. Children and mothers crept towards her, saying, 'What's the time, Mr Wolf?', and when the answer was 'dinner time!' the therapist chased the children, encouraging mothers to hide them in their body shapes. It was found that the mothers who in reality failed to protect their children also failed to protect them in the game, either by letting them stride boldly up to the 'wolf' and/or by failing to contain the children in their body shapes. Children were never 'caught' by the 'wolf', and the therapist was careful to 'de-role' after each game.

7 As the group progressed, less and less structure was used, and the therapist allowed the group members to follow their own impulses, intervening only when it seemed necessary to maintain the aims of the group towards more adaptive functioning. Mothers were encouraged to follow the focus of their child. From time to time, the therapist would also mirror the action, when it seemed appropriate. The main aim of the therapist at this point was to lead as little as possible, yet support the interactional dance between mother and child.

8 In addition to the group sessions, each whole family was offered one or two home sessions. The aim was to integrate the work into the family system, and to attempt to offset any negative effects on the system by the preferential treatment of any one family member; during the pilot study there had been no such policy, and for one family the 'problem' appeared to be transferred from one child to another following DMT with the mother and the identified child (Meekums 1988).

Each session began as group members were collected by the therapist in a minibus and taken to the Unit. Once at the Unit, mothers and children separated for half an hour of DMT, each sub-group being facilitated by either the dance movement therapist or her trainee. There followed half an hour as a group, after which the children played with a volunteer, whilst parents watched a replay of video material from the session. The group then had lunch together, cleared up, and all mothers and children were taken home by minibus.

There follows a recording of session ten, half-way through the DMT programme:

Mothers (facilitated by a trainee)

Aims:
1 Relaxation
2 Use of eye focus
3 Contact
4 Rhythmic synchrony.

Content: Breathing whilst lying on back, rolling heads and leading movement with nose, introducing peripheral vision, walking on counts of eight, using eye contact, massage.
Music: 'Holding Back the Years', 'Run the World'.
Comments: Some embarrassment from the mothers when walking with eye contact. Needed more time.

Children (facilitated by the dance movement therapist)

Aims:
1 To respond to the children
2 To begin to develop child-initiated themes towards a sense of co-operation.

Music: None.
Content: Running and falling on large cushions, 'ring o' roses', forward rolls and helping the dance therapist to roll by pushing her, chasing in a circle, falling down, throwing and catching a ball using the therapist as a focal point.
Comments: The activity flowed much more easily than previous sessions; the two youngest children were distracted by video equipment but easily encouraged back into the group.

Mothers and children (facilitated by the dance movement therapist)

Aim: To provide opportunities for mother–child interaction.
Content: Various activities, arising from the instruction to the mothers that they take their cue from their child. The 'I love you' song to finish, first holding in dyads then as a large group, women linking arms around backs in a circle as the children sat on a cushion.
Music: Various.
Comments: Group functioning almost autonomously, the therapist leading very little but providing a holding role. Mothers now say proper goodbyes to children before separating for initial sections. Some

polarization: two of the women on their feet with their children, bouncy, rhythmically engaged with the music, lots of synchrony; the other two sitting with children on their laps, throwing balls. After a while, this second sub-group picked up on the theme of the first.

The 'I love you' song, adapted from a Sufi song, became a hallmark of the group. Each mother would sit with her child cradled in her arms, making eye contact, and sing:

> I love you, whether I know it or not,
> I love you, whether I show it or not,
> There are so many things I haven't said inside my heart,
> Perhaps now is a good time to start.

CASE ILLUSTRATIONS

In this section, the case studies for two contrasting dyads will be presented: Angela and Alvin (dyad A); and Doreen and Darren (dyad D).[4]

The results of the pilot study (Meekums 1988) suggested that some improvement appears to occur in the mother–child relationship following DMT, when the family system contains other more normally functioning relationships, and there is a history of 'bonding failure' for that pair, for example due to long separations during the first year of life or ambivalence during the pregnancy. These criteria held for Angela and Alvin, and so the prognosis could be said to be good for these two. The existence of sexual abuse in the family of dyad D, however, and the emergence during DMT of the fact that Doreen had herself been sexually abused as a child, and had an unstable relationship with Darren's father, did not offer a good prognosis for Doreen and Darren (see, for example, Kempe and Kempe 1978). The dance movement therapist/researcher did not make any prognosis at the outset, and this analysis has been done retrospectively. It is therefore unlikely that prejudiced views affected the results in this way.

The women were interviewed four times: prior to the start of the DMT programme; half-way through the programme; within one week of the end; and at a six-month follow-up. The pilot study had generated questions concerning:

1 which personal factors, if any, are associated with positive change in mother–child interaction following DMT and therefore what is an appropriate referral;
2 the mother's perception of which aspects of her interaction with her child change most following DMT, and which least;
3 the mother's perceptions of DMT and of the dance movement therapist;

4 which movement behaviours can be observed to change along with the mother's perception of improved interaction with her child.

Information was therefore sought during the initial interview regarding:

1 personal factors, for example whether the mother had been 'in care' as a child;
2 difficulties in the relationship with her child;
3 the mother's goals for change.

During later interviews, the mother's perceptions were sought regarding:

1 the relationship, with particular reference to areas of concern identified at the outset;
2 any changes in the family as a whole;
3 the DMT group and its leaders (the dance movement therapist and a trainee);
4 any other factors which might have affected outcome.

Interviews were conducted by the dance movement therapist/ researcher. The limitation of this combined role is acknowledged. Due to the pioneering nature of this work in Britain, it was not possible to find another experienced practitioner who was in a position to carry out either the interviews or the DMT practice. In recognition that the dance therapist/researcher would have a higher investment in the therapy 'succeeding', a second interviewer was used for a short time during the pilot study (Meekums 1988). The result was that shorter, less informative replies were obtained. There was no evidence that the respondents were trying to please the interviewer because she was the dance movement therapist. In fact quite the contrary: when asked for their honest feelings about the group leaders, they were at times quite critical. On the whole, respondents were more revealing about the extent of their problems in relating to their children as therapy progressed, and the problems had begun to ease. It is therefore possible that the combined role may have facilitated more honest responses from the mothers, since a therapist/client relationship had been built during DMT. However, it is also possible that this relationship was stronger with some mothers than with others.

Each session was recorded in two files: a group file, which was used to record attendance, interventions, and group process; and one individual file (open for the mother to see and comment on) for each dyad, recording casual conversations and details of mother–child interaction, from memory. Movement observation was also carried out retrospectively for each dyad, from video recordings, with reference to the literature on mother–child interaction, and non-verbal communication in families. Of particular importance in determining observation categories was the work of Dulicai (1977).

Angela and Alvin

Angela and Alvin (dyad A) were referred by their social worker, who was closing her work with the family and recommended that they did not need further social work involvement. Alvin, of mixed white and Afro-Caribbean parentage, was the second of three children, and aged 3 years at the start of the DMT programme. Angela was 34 years old, white, and a lone parent; she related well to her youngest child, a girl.

Alvin's older brother had been 'out of control' in the past, after which Alvin appeared to have taken on that role, and was now seen by Angela as the naughtiest in the family. During the social worker's involvement, Angela and Alvin had experienced some 'holding therapy', which necessitated Angela holding Alvin for quite long periods, often against his will. The philosophy of 'holding therapy' conflicted with that of DMT in this context, which made use of holding to convey positive feelings, and not usually against the child's will. Alvin did not like being held, and Angela felt unable to control his behaviour, but appeared to be highly motivated to change the situation.

In the initial interview, Angela said that the main problem was Alvin's 'whinging' and disobedience ('not listening' to her). She complained that he was only happy when the centre of attention. Angela described Alvin as a 'cry baby'. Interestingly, she said that she had been upset during the pregnancy, one minute wanting the baby, another not. She herself never cried in front of the children, because, she said, whenever her own mother had cried it was after she had been beaten by Angela's step-father.

Once in the DMT group, one of the immediately striking aspects of Angela's behaviour was that she tended to shout even the simplest of instructions to her son. She described herself as 'on edge', for which she took both prescribed and non-prescribed medication. She said she ate for comfort, and her weight fluctuated with the swings of bingeing and dieting.

Despite the difficulties described by both Angela and her social worker, some degree of attunement between Angela and Alvin was evident in the early sessions: Angela echoed Alvin's postural shifts, a phenomenon associated by Scheflen (1964) with mutual identification between adults, and in dancing together they showed a high degree of synchrony, subtly exchanging the leadership role as they mirrored each other's shapes and rhythms. However, Angela would at times 'disconnect' from her son, apparently ceasing to be aware of where he was, blocking his access to her, or not meeting him at his level. There was little moulding, and they displayed few affectionate gestures to each other. Their interaction seemed decidedly 'on–off'.

As the group progressed, Angela displayed a growing repertoire for controlling Alvin's behaviour, and on one occasion she also allowed herself to protect him with her body, when he ran from the dance movement therapist who was dancing spikey, witch-like movements.

However, whenever Angela held Alvin she would tend to use disproportionately strong force. She seemed to fight hard in her efforts to control him. It is possible that Alvin felt overpowered rather than supported by this, and the dance movement therapist hypothesized that the key to his 'out-of-control' behaviour lay in this dynamic. At this stage, interventions concentrated on encouraging Angela to adopt positions which facilitated eye contact and on providing opportunities for rhythmic interaction, in which the pair functioned synchronously.

In the children's DMT section, Alvin contributed with original movement ideas. He also showed an increasing willingness to share objects with other children.

Towards approximately the seventh session, the therapist was able to encourage Angela to soften her hold on Alvin and allow him a degree of exploration. She also encouraged Angela to move towards Alvin in order to attract his attention, rather than sit and shout. Angela began to accommodate to Alvin's level. On one occasion, when throwing a ball between them, Angela became very animated, encouraging Alvin with applause, and shouts of 'Again! Yeah!'.

Around this time, a family session was conducted in the home. Alvin regressed to acting out, attention seeking, and being uncooperative. He exaggerated a pattern observed during the sessions, of using his body as a human missile, charging into people and hurting them. The dance movement therapist coined the term 'missiling' for this behaviour, having seen it before in children from a similar population. Angela was shouting more than ever during the home session, resisting suggestions of a quieter approach, claiming that it would not work.

However, in the next group session Angela's control was more effective; she responded with fluidity, rather than battling, and used her own body to softly contain Alvin. The therapist encouraged this trend, suggesting that when Alvin next ran off (as he frequently did) Angela maintain her awareness of him, whilst playing on her own with a ball. The result was that Angela began to use more indulging, nurturing movement qualities (Laban 1960; Ostrov 1981): her voice softened, her shape widened, and her movements became lighter. When Alvin saw her like this, he immediately came to her, and they began to move with the ball together.

In the second interview, half-way through the DMT programme, Angela reported that Alvin had previously tended to stay in a corner at home, but was no longer exhibiting this behaviour. She also said that he now asked first before taking things and was less whingy. She reported that she was more able to make physical contact with him. At this stage, there were no known changes in their external circumstances which could have contributed to the change, other than DMT.

Angela and Alvin's interaction in the sessions continued to become more adaptive. On one occasion, before separating from Alvin for the smaller group sessions, Angela squatted down, holding Alvin's hands, making eye contact, and gently explained, 'When I do some dancing, you do some dancing, then we all do some when I come back'. She then hugged her son, their shapes moulding with each other. On another occasion, Angela spontaneously crawled to Alvin, resulting in more hugs. Alvin then rolled away, and instead of trying to hold onto him, Angela mirrored the roll. Angela seemed to be developing the ability to 'track' her son without having to physically hold him, and hardly ever blocked his access to her now. However, she would still at times intrude on his personal space, which resulted in him pushing her away.

Displays of affection, including stroking and kissing, developed between Angela and Alvin. When another of the children bit Alvin one day, Angela supported and protected Alvin with her body, moulding her body round his, stroking him, rocking, and speaking to him softly. She opened her body shape to allow the children to 'make up', then re-affirmed her support by returning to a moulded shape, and rocking. Although Angela still tended to 'fight' with Alvin, she responded quickly to intervention, defusing potentially explosive situations.

Then Alvin had an ear operation, and Angela appeared to be making excuses not to come to the group. In session fifteen, no one attended the group. This coincided with the removal into local authority care of Doreen's children, and almost certainly reflected a systemic reaction to that loss.

After sensitive communication by the dance movement therapist, Angela and Alvin returned the following week, though Angela saw Alvin as being fragile, and said she must not hit him. Angela rarely hit Alvin in the group, but the removal of this form of discipline was causing her considerable strain. Alvin knew that he must not be hit, and appeared to be pushing for limits to be set. At one point, Alvin hit his mother hard in the face. Angela smacked him hard on the wrist, several times, then pushed him away, shouting 'Get away from me!' Several times, Alvin returned to her, looking bewildered and concerned, only to be pushed away again. Eventually, Angela rushed out of the room, in tears.

The therapist stayed with Alvin, rocking and reassuring him, whilst the trainee counselled Angela. They eventually returned, Angela still in tears, and Angela told Alvin how hurt and upset she felt, asking him never to do it again. He agreed, and the incident concluded with most of the group in tears as the pair cuddled and rocked, telling each other 'I love you'.

Angela repeated her 'I love you' the following week when, blindfolded, she was able to identify Alvin's face. She lightly stroked his cheek, warmly smiled at him, and gently patted his bottom.

In the penultimate session, Angela was in crisis once more; her sister had stolen some of her money, and Angela was rejecting the children, pleading for social work help. Although the therapist thought that this might be at least to some degree a reaction to the impending loss of the group, her plea for help was taken seriously and investigated. However, in the last session Angela acknowledged that she was coping with her crisis, and did not need a social worker. During a trust exercise, she allowed herself to experience the support of the group.

At the interview immediately after the end of the DMT programme, Angela said that Alvin was now whinging only occasionally, and was 'listening' to her more, which was probably at least in part due to his improved hearing following the successful ear operation. Angela said, 'Alvin gets upset if I shout but he never answers me back now'. He was also beginning to take his turn for attention in the family. Angela was much happier:

> We can act about a lot more without him being so miserable . . . I don't feel depressed like I used to – at one time I'd wish for his dad to come and take him away for the weekend – not now.

Angela seemed to be more in control, and more protective towards the children, although she still tended to explode in temper. The two boys were now fighting less, and Angela was insisting that they stay inside the garden to play now, whereas she revealed that she used to let them wander. On the subject of physical closeness, Angela said, 'He'll come and give me a cuddle without me asking . . . if I ask him to sit near me he'll do it – at one time he'd run off.'

She also said that her older son was letting her cuddle him, whereas he would not do so before. Her general comments about the DMT group were:

> I didn't think it'd be any good really. Alvin would enjoy dancing but there'd be nothing for me, or us. I never thought things would change at all . . . [but] I've got more out of the dance group than I have with anybody – my kids are more loving towards me. I feel as if they are mine now, rather than just come out of the world. They can talk to me without me snapping – I can explain to them, which I learned from the dance group . . . I was upset to leave at the end.

At the second follow-up interview six months later, Angela reported that all the improvements were maintained. She continued to speak positively of the DMT group, and was unable to identify anything she disliked about it. She said, 'I miss it more than owt'.[5]

Doreen and Darren

Doreen and an older child had attended a previous group based on DMT principles, led by the current dance movement therapist's predecessor. Darren was the second of three children. The names of all of the children had been previously placed on the 'at risk' register following sexual abuse of the oldest child, a girl. Darren was aged 2 years at the start of the DMT programme, and Doreen was 22 years old. Both were white. Doreen and Darren were referred to the 'Love Bugs' by their social worker, who said that they lacked any personal time together, and Darren did not receive as much attention as his sisters. He was also used as a messenger between his parents during arguments; his father had been known to be violent to his mother. The social worker's expectations were that Doreen would gain from social contact with other women, and would herself be supportive. However, the social worker's expectations of a positive therapeutic outcome for Doreen's relationship with Darren were probably low, although this was not explicitly stated to the dance movement therapist/researcher and so it is unlikely that this view affected the outcome. Unlike the referral of Angela and Alvin, there was little discussion of any goals for the mother's interaction with her child; these seemed to be a less open agenda between social worker and mother, possibly due to the mother's low motivation for personal change.

Doreen revealed at her initial interview that she had been 'in care' as a child; it later transpired that she had been sexually abused. Doreen claimed that Darren was stubborn; she said he tended to stand and scream if he could not get his own way. This was not evident later in the DMT sessions; in fact, Darren displayed extreme passivity. He was also portrayed by Doreen as hitting his 1-year-old sister and fighting with his 4½-year-old sister. However, Doreen did say that when she was alone with him, he was 'no trouble'.

Doreen's depressed body attitude was evident from the outset: her characteristic position was sitting, with her forearms or elbows resting on her knees, and her head either on her arms or in her hands. This position effectively cut Darren out. Her attempts to make contact with him were either weak and ineffectual or sudden and strong. She hardly ever looked directly at him. Darren also looked depressed: his torso was passively heavy but inflexible, and he had a small kinesphere, or sphere of action. He avoided eye contact with the therapist. Darren showed little tendency to follow or be near Doreen.

At the first session, Doreen said that she had left her husband, and had a new boyfriend. But by the next session she was again living with her husband. She also had her arm in a sling. Darren ran off frequently, so the therapist modelled methods of gaining Darren's attention, which were received unenthusiastically by Doreen. Doreen and Darren displayed little synchrony with each other during the DMT sessions, and Doreen frequently blocked Darren's process, for example by taking a prop from him before he could use it. She also blocked his access to her for protection during the game 'What's the time, Mr Wolf?'.

In session three, there appeared to be some progress. Doreen began to respond to Darren, to cuddle and kiss and praise, and the angry words became fewer. When he ran off, Doreen distracted Darren with a game. Darren emerged from his passive state a little, and even suggested playing 'ring o' roses'. At around this time, Doreen formed an alliance with another young woman in the group. She said that she wanted another baby now that she was reunited with her husband, and the following week Doreen announced that pregnancy was a possibility. The positive interactions continued, Darren began to look more alive, his speech improved, and he began to accept limits from Doreen. They even made eye contact across the room on one occasion, and Doreen made some attempts to position herself at Darren's level.

The pregnancy was confirmed by session five, and Doreen began to talk about her daughter's sexual abuse, in the past tense. She began to take more care of Darren, holding him in the minibus to make him safe.

But when the dance movement therapist facilitated the children's section in session seven, she observed that Darren did not respond to pain in the usual way. He only whimpered a little when bitten hard by one of the other children. Compared to the other children Darren still seemed lethargic, always tired, hardly ever smiling. He hid behind pieces of furniture, and did not assert his right to hold onto the ball, although, once offered it, he seemed to enjoy throwing and kicking. However, his use of weight appeared to be increasing a little, as was his kinesphere.

Doreen displayed a pattern of blocking Darren's access to her at the beginning of each session, gradually facilitating access as the session progressed. When working with an object, she tended to put her own impulses first, rather than facilitate Darren's. She also still tended to 'lose track' of him in the room.

At the second interview, the dance movement therapist/researcher emphasized the gains made in the sessions, and Doreen admitted for the first time that she had tended to exclude Darren at home, though she said she did this less now. She also felt that her oldest daughter was benefiting from ripple effects in the family, but Doreen was concerned about the £20 owed to her by one of the other mothers, which was causing friction in the group.

Doreen began to seek out the trainee for chats. She was feeling nauseous by session eight, and was understandably less vigilant when Darren ran off. However, they were able to relate through a ball, rolling it between them and copying various movements.

By session nine, Darren was no longer hiding during the children's section, though he was unable to 'catch' a ball, even when it was placed in his hands. At one point he rolled back and forth on the ball, in a quasi-sexual rhythm. On that day, Doreen had left her older daughter in the care of a man who had been suspected of sexually abusing her. The dance movement therapist became concerned about the children's protection.

In view of this concern, and Darren's problems in using his weight to assert himself, the dance movement therapist began working with Darren, using hand to hand contact, and asking him to 'push' her over. No matter how little effort he used, the therapist fell over each time, then bounced back and encouraged him to repeat the action, pushing harder. Gradually his response increased, though it remained weak. Doreen was encouraged to take over the dance movement therapist's role, which she did, though she fell less easily. Perhaps by coincidence, or perhaps because of the mobilization of Darren's weight, Darren began to say 'no' in the following session. He began to stand his ground, rather than running away.

The next task for the therapist was to acknowledge Darren's pain when hurt. When this was mentioned to Doreen, she said that Darren's father tended to laugh at him when he was hurt. Darren had learned to laugh at his own pain, and had recently laughed when he had cut his head, until he saw the blood, when he screamed. The confusion of pain and pleasure was communicated to the social worker, and the question raised of possible sexual abuse, though this remained speculation. The dance movement therapist continued the work on Darren's push response.

Darren continued to develop in the children's section, dancing a delightful twirl, and displaying a new sense of his expanding kinesphere. Vestiges of moulding appeared between Doreen and Darren, but progress remained minimal. On one occasion, Doreen was in her characteristic closed-off position when the dance movement therapist asked her if she was all right. She answered that she was playing a game with Darren. In fact, Darren was not engaged in the game, but was lying on the floor in isolation.

Doreen tended to prod and poke at Darren, and put him down abruptly, like a sack of potatoes that was too heavy to carry. She would sometimes initiate dance movements for Darren to follow, but did not tend to echo his movements. When playing ball with another pair, Doreen sat behind Darren, gripping his wrists, and using his body like a puppet to throw and catch the ball. When Darren tried to wriggle free, Doreen pulled him back sharply. Darren's resistance to Doreen was in contrast to his smile as the ball approached.

At the home session, Doreen was observed picking up her youngest daughter by the wrists, from behind. The dance movement therapist modelled the appropriate behaviour (*en face*, holding round the torso), but with little effect. Darren seemed lively, but when he hit his head, as he tended to regularly both in and out of DMT sessions, he became very still and looked 'glazed' for a whilst. Some quasi-sexual behaviour was observed; when playing a game in which one child is swung and held by the arms and legs by two adults (initiated by Doreen), the youngest girl repeatedly tapped the genitals of the oldest girl, who laughed. The dance movement therapist noted this interaction, but did not intervene during the session as the behaviour may have been indicative of normal development; it did not seem appropriate to mention this behaviour to the mother in front of the children, as this may have given them the impression that they were in some way 'bad'; to have mentioned it later would have been to exaggerate its potential importance at that time, or to risk loss of trust.

In the following session, twelve, Darren cried when he hurt himself during the children's section. He also used his arms to protect himself by breaking his fall as he came down a slide. These were seen as positive developments. Once again, Doreen said that she was splitting up from her husband, but he was still in the family home. The children had all witnessed a fight between their parents. The potential break-up coincided with the impending loss of Doreen's social worker and thoughts about the group coming to an end.

By session fourteen, the father had still not left, and Darren presented with a cut on his hand, which Doreen said had been due to the father leaving his razor on the side of the bath. When Darren began head-banging, Doreen said that her oldest child also did this. Doreen seemed especially caring to Darren.

The cut was routinely reported to the social worker. When Darren attended a children's group at LFSU later that week, he told the playgroup worker that 'Daddy had cut him', and that he had 'hurt him in bed'. A paediatrician found evidence of recent anal abuse in the oldest child, who disclosed that her father had anally abused both herself and Darren. There was a cigarette burn on the youngest child. A place of safety order was taken, and access strictly limited. Doreen returned to the group once alone before it ended.

Because of the sensitive situation, Doreen was not asked questions about herself and Darren at the interview immediately after the end of the DMT programme. About the group, she said she felt shy at first, but angry that it had ended:

> It gave me time to get out of the house and let myself go . . . I felt easier with [the trainee]; she didn't nag at me with Darren. You used to say 'go back and get Darren's coat' [when it was cold]; I used to get mad if you'd caught me on a bad morning.

The six-month follow-up was omitted for Doreen or Darren, since all three children were still 'in care'.

CONCLUSIONS

Cohn and Daro (1987), in their analysis of a large number of evaluation studies concerning therapeutic interventions with abused children and their families, found that more than one-third of parents mistreated their children during treatment, and more than half were judged likely to do so following treatment. In this author's research study, similar outcomes were obtained. Only dyad A showed a sufficient improvement in mother–child interaction to no longer need social work help, and dyad D was evidently part of a family in which abuse occurred during the DMT programme.

The two most consistent factors associated with the development of positive mother–child interaction appear to have been:

1 the presence of other more adaptive mother–child relationships in the family;
2 evidence of previous interruption in the attachment process for the mother and child being studied.

This was true both for dyad A and one other, dyad C, whose case is not presented here but who also made some progress in their relationship during DMT. It may therefore be reasonably concluded that an appropriate referral to group DMT for mothers and young children at risk of abuse might be made when these two factors are present. However, maternal motivation appears also to be a significant factor; although neither Angela (dyad A) nor the mother in dyad C believed initially that the therapy would 'work', the aims were clearly explained and goals agreed at the outset, implying that these two women were open to DMT, and both mothers viewed the DMT and the therapist positively by the end of the programme. These mothers were also the two oldest in the group, and it is possible that their maturity facilitated their acceptance of DMT.

Negative outcome appears to have been associated with the mother's own history of abuse for dyad D, and this is consistent with Kempe and Kempe (1978). It is possible that, if individual DMT had been available for the mother, this factor might have become insignificant. It is also possible that the small amount of direct work with Darren that occurred during the DMT programme facilitated his disclosure; there is no conclusive evidence for this, but the outcome, whilst negative in terms of mother–child interaction, was positive in that it resulted in protection for Darren and his siblings. This also points to the relevance of individual work with children whose families contain multiple dysfunction. It is possible that DMT has a role to play in disclosure and therapeutic work with children for whom there is a suspicion of sexual abuse, since the approach places some emphasis on the development of appropriate body boundaries, and on issues of personal power and control. However, in working with any one part of the family system, the effects on the whole should be borne in mind; to work with a child who is still living in a hostile environment might be to put her or him at greater risk; from negative reactions by adults to growing assertion by the child, for example.

The degree of positive change evident in the research study (Meekums 1990) appears to have been unrelated to the kind of birth experienced, the size of the family, or position of the child in that family. However, the older children like Alvin seem to have fared best. It may be that these children's maturity enabled them to respond to their mothers' attention during the group in such a way that their mothers did not perceive them as clingy, but rewarding.

There was a marked similarity in the reports obtained during the research study, particularly at the interview immediately after the end of the DMT programme, from the mothers of the two dyads who made most progress (dyads A and C). Both reported: an increase in cuddles; better control of the child's behaviour; feeling closer to the child; improved communication, including verbal; more positive behaviour by the child towards her; an initial disbelief that the group would 'work'; positive feelings about the group at the end, and sadness that it had ended. In addition they felt that they were helped by the therapist sharing her own problems on one or two occasions; that there were improved relationships with other children in the family system; and that they appreciated the therapist's direct interventions to assist change in dysfunctional interactional behaviours, though one woman admitted she had not always liked it at the time. This last point contrasts strongly with the reports of the two women for whom less positive change was noted (from dyads B and D), and who were younger. Both preferred the trainee/co-worker, who was younger than the therapist, and was less direct in her interventions.

Although similar to findings of Payne (1988), and Jordan (1988), an increase in verbal communication was not one of the aims of the DMT programme. One possible explanation for this result is that the mothers had to explain activities to their children, and so the channels of verbal communication were opened. However, few explanations by the mothers to their children were necessary during the DMT programme; the emphasis was more on improvisation than on structured activity, and so this explanation of the result does not appear to hold.

One other possible explanation is that the 'concept of the dialogue' (Schaffer 1977), in other words the reciprocal give and take evident in a conversation, was utilized in movement interactions, and provided the basis for later verbal interaction, following the developmental sequence of a mother and her infant. If this is the case, and it remains unproven, DMT may have a role in developing language for children with a range of learning and other difficulties. It could be argued that the development of verbal communication was simply due to maturation. However, if this were so, it might have been reported in cases which had a less favourable outcome overall; this was not the case. The issues concerning language acquisition are complex, and any attempts at explanation of this result remain speculative. Further research is needed to throw light on the relationship between DMT and language acquisition, for example through controlled studies involving assessments of language development in groups of children receiving either DMT or gymnastics.

Another feature of the process was the gradual disclosure by the mothers of the extent of their difficulties with their children. Such a process is entirely understandable; at the outset, to admit to not loving one's child must be both painful and frightening, and the fear of judgement, or of perhaps losing the child, must be an important factor. With the development of the therapeutic alliance between each mother and the dance movement therapist, disclosure becomes easier. Such a process makes any attempt to standardize data from interviews extremely hazardous, and forces the researcher also to pursue other means of enquiry. The importance of the development of trust in facilitating disclosure illustrates the unique nature of each DMT intervention; the therapist and the therapy are inseparable, part of an interacting system. It is also possible that the use of a non-verbal therapy assisted the mother's verbal disclosure, providing a route to difficult and painful feelings or memories that might not have been easily accessed by verbal means alone.

It is possible that the DMT provided opportunities for positive interaction, and that these interactions, along with verbal encouragement from the dance movement therapist, constituted a reward, thus reinforcing the behaviour. If so, one could expect that the interactions would be returned to again and again. Indeed, some repetition was observed during the improvisations, from one week to the next. Repeated movement sequences often involved mirroring '*en face*' or moulded 'gee-gee' rides on all fours. Systems of reward imply a behaviourist approach to therapy, which is generally assumed to have little in common with DMT (BBernstein 1979), although meaningful social interaction is seen as one of the goals of DMT, and this may at times include specific focus on new ways of responding (Bernstein 1979). It could also be argued that in the context of children at risk of abuse there is little time to enter into lengthy, in-depth therapy. The results of the author's research pointed to the need for a flexible approach to DMT, the methods being defined by the population and setting.

The finding that some mothers were helped by the therapist's disclosure of her own problems on one or two occasions is consistent with the reported findings of Prodgers and Bannister (1983) in their dramatherapy work with mothers of abused children. The usefulness of carefully controlled revelations might lie in the development of trust, and the 'therapeutic alliance'; effectively, the mother views the therapist as being 'on her side'. This finding also supports the view that the therapist and the therapy are inseparable.

From the author's research, the movement observation categories found to be associated with positive outcome were: echoing or synchrony; moulding; and access to the mother's body.

Those associated with negative outcome were: partial body actions, which inhibit moulding; blocking of eye contact by the child; and the child resisting the mother's movement initiations.

An unexpected increased tendency in all dyads for the mother to block the child's explorations was noted. The increase was smallest in those for whom a positive outcome was noted, and may have been insignificant in these cases; it was greatest in dyad D (the most negative outcome). The behaviour may have signalled the higher degree of control being exerted by each mother over her child's behaviour, although it is possible that for dyad D the high level of blocking was indicative of dysfunction. Darren displayed an increased resistance to Doreen's initiations, and her greatly increased attempts to control him may have been due to non-acceptance of this growing assertion. It is possible that greater parental control, exhibited by blocking of the child's process, is adaptive in the formation of clear boundaries up to a certain threshold. This might be particularly expected when the mother has previously complained that her child is disobedient. However, it is possible that beyond a certain point the tendency becomes maladaptive, which appears to have been the case for dyad D. Clearly, the issue is complex, and any interpretation of the data must remain at the level of conjecture, until or unless further research throws more light on the relationships between blocking of the child's explorations, child abuse, and the development of appropriate boundaries during DMT.

The changes observed in movement behaviour are consistent with Dulicai (1977), whose research indicated that normally functioning families display more moulding and full body actions, as well as fewer static body attitudes than dysfunctional families. The association between echoing or synchrony and the development of positive mother–child relationships is consistent with Condon and Sander (1974), Fraenkel (1983), Schaffer (1977), and Stern (1971, 1977). The significance of moulding, a spatial phenomenon, and echoing or synchrony, which are both temporal and spatial phenomena, is also consistent with Winnicott's (1960) suggestion that the holding environment is initially spatial, becoming temporal. Because moulding, echoing, and synchrony are behaviours associated with early mother–child movement behaviour, the possibility thus arises that DMT can specifically address the essence of early mother–child interaction, and thus the building blocks of mother–child attachment. Silberstein (1984) has suggested that moulding is associated primarily with attachment behaviours between mothers and young children. Further research is needed to establish clearly the developmental significance of moulding and echoing, for example in DMT with larger samples of mothers and children of differing ages.

ACKNOWLEDGEMENTS

I wish to thank Mrs P. Sanderson of the University of Manchester; Ms D. Dulicai, ADTR, of Hahnemann University USA; and the staff, management, and consumers of Leeds Family Service Unit for their help in this project. The practice was made possible by a grant from the Headley Trust and some financial assistance was received for the research study from both LFSU and the Sir Richard Stapeley Trust.

NOTES

1 The term 'holding environment' is used by Winnicott (1965) to mean both the way that a mother holds the infant and the general attitude of the mother (which affects her behaviour) of bearing the baby in mind as a whole person and protecting the child from traumatic impingement from the environment, which might cause her or him to react and experience a break in a sense of continuity of being.
2 In this chapter, the term 'mother' is used to denote the primary care-giver, whether male or female, except when referring to the sample. In this context, all of the mothers were women.
3 Here, interactional synchrony implies dyadic movements which begin at precisely the same time, whereas echoing implies a staggered onset.
4 All names of participants in the DMT programme have been changed.
5 'Owt' is Yorkshire vernacular for 'anything'.

REFERENCES

Bell, J. (1984) 'Family therapy in motion: observing, assessing and changing the family dance', in P. Lewis (ed.) *Theoretical Approaches in Dance-Movement Therapy*, Vol. 2, Dubuque, IA: Kendall/Hunt.

Cohn, A. and Daro, D. (1987) 'Is treatment too late: what ten years of evaluative research tell us', *Child Abuse and Neglect* 11: 433–42.

Condon, W. S. (1968) 'Linguistic-kinesic research and dance therapy', *Proceedings of 3rd Annual Conference of the ADTA*.

Condon, W. and Sander, L. (1974) 'Neonate movement is synchronized with adult speech: interactional participation and language acquisition', *Science (USA)* 183: 99–101.

Dulicai, D. (1977) 'Nonverbal assessment of family systems: a preliminary study', *Art Psychotherapy* 4: 55–68.

Fraenkel, D. (1983) 'The relationship of empathy in movement to synchrony, echoing, and empathy in verbal interactions', *American Journal of Dance Therapy* 6: 31–48

Graham, C. (1984) 'The use of dance and movement therapy as a social work technique', unpublished dissertation submitted in part fulfilment of Master of Social Work, University of York.

Jordan, L. (1988) 'Dance for the handicapped: a comparison between the aims and objectives of the dance therapist and the dance educationalist', unpublished dissertation submitted in part fulfilment of M. Ed., University of Manchester.

Kempe, R. and Kempe, C. H. (1978) *Child Abuse*, London: Fontana.

Kestenberg, J. (1975) *Children and Parents: Psychoanalytic Studies in Development*, New York: Jason Aronson.

Kestenberg, J. and Buelte, A. (1977) 'Prevention, infant therapy and the treatment of adults: 2. Mutual holding and holding oneself up', *International Journal of Psychoanalytic Psychotherapy* 6: 369–96.

Laban, R. Von (1960) *The Mastery of Movement*, second edition, London: Macdonald & Evans.

Lewis, P. (1979) 'A holistic frame of reference in dance-movement therapy' in P. Lewis (ed.) *Theoretical Approaches in Dance-Movement Therapy*, Vol 1, Dubuque, IA: Kendall/Hunt.

Meekums, B. (1988) 'Dance movement therapy and the development of mother–child interaction – a pilot study', *Proceedings of Dance and the Child International Conference*, Roehampton Institute, London.

——(1990) 'Dance movement therapy and the development of mother–child interaction', unpublished M.Phil. thesis, University of Manchester.

Murphy, J. (1979) 'The use of non-verbal and body movement techniques in working with families with infants', *Journal of Marital and Family Therapy* October: 61–6.

Ostrov, K. (1981) 'A movement approach to the study of infant/caregiver communication during infant psychotherapy', *American Journal of Dance Therapy* 4(1): 25–41.

Payne, H. (1988) 'The use of dance movement therapy with troubled youth', in C. E. Schaefer (ed.) *Innovative Interventions in Child and Adolescent Therapy*, New York, London, Sydney: Wiley Interscience, pp. 68–97.

Prodgers, A. and Bannister, A. (1983) 'Actions speak louder than words', *Community Care* July 28: 22–3.

Schaffer, R. (1977) *Mothering*, London: Open Books.

Scheflen, A. E. (1964) 'The significance of posture in communication systems', *Psychiatry* 27: 316–24.

Silberstein, S. (1984) 'Expressive movement in children and mothers: focus on individuation', in D. Dulicai and S. Silberstein (eds) *The Arts in Psychotherapy* 11: 63–8.

Stern, D. (1971) 'A micro-analysis of mother–infant interaction', *Journal of American Academy of Child Psychiatry* 10(3): 501–16.

——(1977) *The First Relationship: Infant and Mother*, London: Open Books.

Webster, J. (1987) 'A comparison of functional and dysfunctional adoptive families: a non-verbal assessment', unpublished dissertation submitted in part fulfilment of Master of Creative Arts in Therapy, Hahnemann University, USA.

Winnicott, D. (1960) 'The theory of the parent–infant relationship', in *The Maturational Processes and the Facilitating Environment*, London: Hogarth Press, 1965, pp. 37–55.

——(1965) *The Maturational Processes and the Facilitating Environment*, London: Hogarth Press.

Chapter 3

Shut in, shut out

Dance movement therapy with children and adolescents

Helen Payne

INTRODUCTION

This chapter is a distillation of reflections over ten years of practice and research in dance movement therapy with children and adolescents in special education. In DMT there is an engagement with bodily movement towards the aim of transformation. This takes place in a symbolic space. Winnicott believes therapy takes place in the overlap of two areas of playing, that of the patient and that of the therapist. This potential play space is that which is between the subjective object and the object which is subjectively perceived. It has to do with 'two people playing together' (Winnicott 1971: 38) and is very much about doing.

In a sense, the stages of childhood and adolescence are also in a transitional time and place, not yet in the mainstream street of life as independent people yet no longer a person fully protected, totally dependent on the pavement of life. (It is ironic that many of the populations referred to in this chapter are very often literally on our streets in a vulnerable condition.) Important changes take place at these stages of growth which build on the foundations of psychological life laid down in infancy. Play is normally a central feature of childhood, as is action. There is often anger as well as love and the imagination plays a central role in relation to inner worlds.

By reading this chapter you will get an idea of the theoretical underpinnings of working in DMT with this population as well as unique insight into the client's experience of DMT.

The chapter is divided into two sections for ease of reading. The first section will give the reader help in understanding the background to working with children and adolescents and an up-to-date survey of research and of those practitioners who have documented in this area. There is a theoretical overview, including a detailed review of the literature, together with a specific focus on adolescence and delinquency.

The second section concentrates on practical application, core concepts, and a case illustration which is based on an adolescent's perceptions of their experience of the DMT process. This is in contrast to other literature where only the therapist's view of the process is reported. By not including the client's experience of the DMT process there is an underlying assumption that it is not of any importance in our study of DMT. I strongly believe that an understanding of the client's reality of the process is crucial to their engaging with the process of change in DMT. One of my research studies explores this aspect of the work in depth (Payne 1986, 1987, 1988a, 1988b).

Finally, the conclusion presents some of the implications of the work and considers the future of DMT with children and adolescents.

I BACKSTAGE

The two distinct contexts for the material presented are those of a) special school settings for those with moderate learning difficulties and autistic/psychotic children and adolescents and b) residential school settings, which include an education centre of a regional community home with education on the premises (CHE) for young people 'in care' for a variety of reasons, particularly for being out of parental control. (This facility is called a List D school in Scotland.) Both settings contain children and adolescents with challenging behaviour, many of whom are considered emotionally disturbed for a variety of reasons. Much of the material is equally applicable to intermediate treatment and psychiatric settings for children and adolescents such as young people's units or child and family psychiatric clinics.

Theoretical introduction

The children and adolescents to which this chapter refers have labels which include emotionally/behaviourally disturbed (EBD), mal-adjusted, delinquent, deprived, disadvantaged, conduct-disordered, learning disabled, autistic, and psychotic. These diagnoses include problems of non-communication, hyperactivity, language impairment, anorexia, school phobia, and depression. There is not the space here to review each of these conditions individually so an overview of the general categories is given. Definitions and references in the literature are connected to accounts and research studies concerned with emotional disturbance/maladjustment; delinquency; autism/ childhood psychosis; and moderate learning difficulties.

Wilson and Evans (1980), in defining the term 'disturbed', refer to it as describing any abnormality of behaviour, emotion, or relationship sufficiently marked or sufficiently prolonged to cause handicap to a child themselves and/or distress or disturbance in the family or community. This would include children who are 'difficult' or 'disruptive' in school whilst having normal relationships in other social groups. This definition has an educational orientation.

The label 'delinquent' is a complex, multi-faceted term applied to a range of children and adolescents who, for varied reasons, present as troubled or troublesome and are brought to the attention of the juvenile justice system. There seems to be an overlap between maladjustment, or E.B.D., emotional/behavioural disturbance, (an educational term), emotional disturbance (a psychological term), and delinquency (a social term). The terms maladjustment and delinquency are used interchangeably depending on the assessors and referring agencies. Evidence seems to show that those presenting with disturbed behaviours are labelled E.B.D., needing help and treatment, until they persistently offend when they are labelled delinquent, needing control if not punishment. Many of those labelled E.B.D. and delinquent are shown to have a learning disability in addition.

The author defines delinquency as being concerned with neglected and disaffected young people who make trouble for themselves and others, who are 'in trouble' and troubled. The DMT work refers to those delinquents who present with anxiety in addition.

Autism is different from those conditions previously described. It is a communication disability, which involves specific impairment in the understanding and use of conversational language, intonation, gesture, facial expression, and other bodily expression. There is a difficulty in social relationships including poor social empathy and a rejection of normal body contact. Other aspects such as ritualistic behaviour, resistance to change, and obsessional behaviour are also manifested. These children often present with challenging behaviour and a severe learning disability. Childhood psychosis is a general term for the more serious forms of emotional suffering. Both of these conditions are handicapping.

Many of those in receipt of education for moderate learning difficulties are in care in the community. They have often experienced a deprived early childhood, and in family crises and breakdowns are placed 'in care' such as fostering. There is usually a high proportion from educational priority areas and many are from large families, often on income support. They are characterized by low self-esteem, low school achievement; they have been assessed by psychologists as below the normal intelligence for mainstream education, and are normally 'statemented', often removed from their peers to attend a special school. Gaps in knowledge are sometimes the result of frequent school placements and/or their inattentiveness. Difficulties in verbal skills, in listening, in play, and their constant restlessness show a need for a reliable relationship with an adult (Holmes 1977, 1983).

The approach

Dance movement therapy is an alternative strategy for treatment for these groups of young people. It is action-based, involving verbal and vocal exchange but not dependent on a high level of language skills. The body and movement are the vehicle for expression and communication in a pre-verbal and symbolic manner. It is dance in so far as the person engaged or observing perceives it to be so. DMT uses dance in many of its manifestations, from the small dance noticed in stillness to the complex, rhythmic, gestural, phrased patterns and steps through space more generally accepted as dance. Symbolism and the use of the body as metaphor are fundamental to the approach. It embraces elements from dance which include rhythm, space, and energy. Creative movement (based on Laban's principles), rather than prescribed steps, is the basis of the approach, although task orientated or developmental movement approaches are also utilized depending on the population. However, it is not a highly prescribed or corrective approach in terms of a remediation programme for body movement or behavioural reform. It serves to involve the young people in a creative, relationship-building experience with the aim of definition of self. Other approaches use this aim as the core of a treatment programme – for example, child and family psychiatry, intermediate treatment, and social services groups.

My training and experience in humanistic, behavioural, and psycho-analytic therapies have enabled the DMT approach to be adapted to the differing populations. For example, group-analytic dance has been found to be inappropriate for low-functioning, non-verbal groups, but with adolescents in psychiatry this approach has been possible. At times the author has found a behavioural approach helpful with autistic children and young offenders. Hence the model has needed to adapt, depending on the needs of the client, and has developed over the years. It was found that with autistic children one to one work was more effective when combined with sessions in small groups. With adolescents labelled delinquent sessions contained the aggression when they were task-centred with movement games or body-orientated competitions, for example, against the self in holding a posture (as used in bioenergetics) or in pairs and small groups within the group. Here the therapist conducted the physical activity in a way which structured their flight and fight issues, whilst enabling a maintenance of their identity. Warm-ups are often simple movement exercises and warm-downs use relaxation methods. Props, role play, and music are prevalent with these groups. However, with younger, latency-aged autistic and some learning disabled children, developmental stages focused the work, for example through the movements of rocking and crawling to sitting. Some groupwork in a circle was also used and for those with a moderate learning difficulty images could be accessed from, for example, movement improvisations or postures (as used in Gestalt therapy). Each of the strategies developed was selected to work with the specific themes emerging from the clients aiming towards the therapeutic goals.

For example, in my group-analytic training group only verbalization was expected. When I attempted to entreat my colleagues in the group to make physical contact this was, naturally, interpreted by one of the conductors[1]. During the two years of these weekly sessions gross physical movement was restricted too, although after the sessions people usually moved around the space a great deal. After the final session, not surprisingly, much physical contact was made when saying our goodbyes to each other. On the wall in that room there was a large picture of Freud, the father of verbal therapy, with his arms folded, staring down upon us. This remains in my memory. It was one of his students, Wilhelm Reich, who took a controversial posture when he developed a therapeutic approach using the body, breath, and physical touch as tools. My approach has been influenced by both these pioneers as well as Jung, and they are drawn upon as appropriate. For example, DMT which uses the circle aiming at ongoing synchronous movement to music may be a useful approach to establish safety and trust in the early stages of the group. However, there are often fewer participation difficulties in group-analytic dance which can be designed to help the more reluctant or disturbed adolescents to invent movement and participate with the whole group (including the conductor). It enhances motivation by involving each member at the same level; adolescents frequently have a fear of being excluded; with this approach no one has to be in the spotlight too long yet all get attention. For those used to using flight (or action) as everyday defences against change, non-action or reflection/verbal interaction reduces their defensiveness and heightens intensity. If the conductor adopts a low profile the efficacy of the approach is less dependent on the personal style of the therapist and reduces issues about authority so prevalent amongst this population. The aim is to work with the individual by means of the group itself (Foulkes 1965; Foulkes and Anthony 1984). Using free-floating group association in movement, sound, and words, an explanation of the group's unconscious is possible where members themselves interpret the processes. In the verbal dialogue following the movement the individual is regarded as the spokesperson for the group as well as for themselves. There needs to be sufficient ego strength and heterogeneity in behaviour for this approach to be sufficiently engaged with by adolescents.

The psychotic child or adolescent is often in an extreme state of permeability in body boundary as they seem to merge with the walls, giving little sense of differentiation of the self. Autistic children often seem overly rigid in their boundaries. Impervious to contact in any way, they seem to separate themselves totally from others. By working with physical contact in DMT the therapist can physically hold the child, enabling a modification of body boundary, as well as holding a space in their mind for the child's feelings. Merging and separation are recurring issues throughout life and have many feelings attached to them; physical contact can become a metaphor for these.

A review of the relevant research and literature

There is a clear relationship between DMT and psychotherapeutic approaches. In educational settings there are few relevant studies of DMT with children and adolescents, so it is of help to look at those in the other arts therapies and psychotherapy. The latter has particular links with DMT which uses many of the concepts and skills found in verbal psychotherapy. Throughout the review reference is made to several UK works, although American material is also cited if thought to be appropriate.

Dance movement therapy

Although much of the literature to date has been published in America where the practice of DMT is more established, not all relevant research and accounts are from there. For example, North (1972) documents her research in movement therapy with maladjusted children and a year later work in a residential school and with deaf children (North 1973). Meier (1979) gives an overview of her work with special needs children. Payne (1981) describes movement therapy in a special school for children and adolescents with learning difficulties, with the emotionally disturbed (Payne 1984), and a research study of DMT with male adolescents labelled delinquent (Payne 1985, 1986, 1987, 1988a, 1988b). Sherborne (1990) gives an updated account of her work in developmental movement with learning disabled children. Billington (1981) describes intensive work based on Sherborne's (1975) techniques in a school for maladjusted boys. Groves (1979) describes dance experiences for girls with moderate learning difficulties.

In an unpublished research study by Scott (1988) an evaluation of the outcomes of dance and movement in the curriculum of EBD children showed that for young offenders in a CHE the dance form of contact improvisation was effective in the national curriculum areas of personal and social education.

There have been some American writings on the use of DMT in education. Early material includes, for example, Tipple (1975) on performance and social skills and Rogers (1977) on a research study which showed that people with higher cognitive ratings showed a greater movement complexity which increased as social skills levels increased.

There have been studies with autistic children (including Kalish 1968; Siegel 1973; Wislochi 1981; Cole 1982) and Leventhal has published widely on her work with learning disabled and emotionally disturbed children (for example, Leventhal 1974, 1980). In a more recent paper Rakusin (1990) has explored the incorporation of movement education concepts into DMT. The author supports the notion in this literature that the non-verbal medium of DMT can be particularly helpful as a form of intervention with those whose verbal ability is limited.

Early descriptive accounts include Delany (1973) on DMT with elementary-aged, emotionally disturbed children in a psycho-educational day hospital. She stresses the importance of movement as a vehicle for the therapeutic relationship. Balaz (1977) and Fisher (1980) explore creative movement with the learning disabled child in education, claiming it affects the body image and self-concept. Fisher stresses that, although structure is important, too much structure, such as imposed exercises, can produce automatic behaviour rather than help the child towards discovery. Adler and Fisher (1984) examine movement integrated with other arts therapies in the promotion of, for example, awareness of self. Creadick (1985), discussing the arts therapies in relation to handicapped children in education, emphasizes that the process of the artistic endeavour is more important than the product. This does imply that there is a desired aesthetic process, which I would not wholly agree is an appropriate outcome for DMT; however, she does suggest that it is how the response is expressed in the body which indicates to the therapist how far the individual has developed physically and psychologically. Wiener and Helbraun (1985) suggest creative movement with the learning disabled child is helpful in the psychophysical development of the child. According to that article, the greater the muscle differentiation the more physically articulated and emotionally communicative become the internal impulses, resulting in a more gratifying experience of moving. Shennum (1987) examined the effect of art and dance/movement therapy on latency-aged children in residential settings, finding a reduction in acting out and a greater level of emotional responsiveness.

Literature supports the notion that there are many social motivations and reinforcers which encourage children and adolescents to dance. In my work there were certain dance crazes such as bodypopping and breakdance which seemed to enable some young people to engage in DMT more easily where testing, particularly of body skills, was present. Other accounts, such as Lovell (1980), suggest that DMT may be significant for use with adolescents because of the particular body-related issues of puberty, helping to resolve body image concerns. Examples include supporting the transition from child to adult by exploring the psychosexual issues relating to body image via movement processes; developing an acceptance of the differences between child and adolescent intrinsic to the adolescent phase of development; increasing awareness of the psychological and physical changes through verbal and non-verbal means; and heightening body awareness through proprioceptive and tactile stimulation. Research studies stress the importance of DMT in the treatment of child sexual abuse, for example, Wheeler (1987), Goodhill (1987), and, in the UK, Meekums (1990).

Dunne et al. (1982) have reported group body therapy approaches with hospitalized adolescents in the UK as reducing sexual behaviour and violence, increasing verbal interaction, and leading to showing deeper concern for each other. However, the authors do not make their approach clear. Berrol (1989) gives an overview of DMT in special education in Israel where referrals were prominently found to be psycho-social. Lasseter et al. (1989) describe the results of DMT given as part of a school counselling programme for multi-disabled adolescents.

More recently Johnson and Eicher (1990) describe how drama exercises can help in enabling adolescents in a psychiatric unit, particularly those with conduct disorders, to take part in DMT. They highlight how adolescent DMT sessions are often structured exercise classes or, at the other extreme, chaotic and disruptive, leading to therapists' frustrations and doubts about their competence.

Some literature focuses on the relief of anxiety in older adolescents in relation to dance/DMT which is important to note. For example, Leste and Rust (1984), in a UK study, explored the effect of modern dance training on levels of anxiety. Findings showed significant reductions in anxiety for the dance group and not for the other groups of sport and music. No obvious reasons were given, but the authors concluded that the effects of music and physical exercise alone were less than when combined in dance. They found that the more interested the subjects were in dance prior to the programme the more favourable were the effects. This implies that the client's attitude towards dance and movement may dictate the degree to which dance (or DMT) might be useful to them.

Early research by Fisher and Cleveland (1968) refers to anxiety tension in psychiatric patients, saying it could be relieved through the use of movement therapy and relaxation sessions. Kearne (1978), in a study with elementary-aged children following movement classes, claimed a reduction in anxiety.

Other studies stress the value of DMT, movement, and dance with children for remediating disabilities. For example, in an early one, Apter *et al.* (1978) used movement therapy for diagnosing, then treating body behaviour with psychotic adolescents; and Hulton (1985), in a UK school project, used movement and words with adolescent learning disabled and maladjusted boys to improve trust, self-exploration, and articulation.

In general, rigorous research in DMT literature with reference to children and adolescents is mostly limited to studies which concentrate on efficacy, as in relation to body image, perceptual motor development, or affective states such as relief of anxiety. There are several descriptive accounts which cover a range of populations in educational and psychiatric settings.

Arts therapies

There is also documentation to show that other arts therapies which have relevance have been applied in educational settings. For example, in art therapy, Dalley (1990) and Case (1981, 1986, 1987, 1990) have described their work in mainstream schools, special education units, and assessment centres.

Music therapy has a long tradition of work with children, particularly the Nordoff and Robbins (1965) approach with the profoundly and severely learning disabled, including autistic children. Juliette Alvin (1966) has successfully integrated her work within the school setting. More recently Bunt (1986), in a research project, refers to turn-taking as an outcome with learning disabled children in nurseries and special schools.

There are accounts of the use of dramatherapy with children and adolescents, beginning with Jennings's (1973) book *Remedial Drama*. Shuttleworth (1981) has documented his work in adolescent psychiatry and Jennings and Gersie (1987) show the potential of dramatherapy in their work.

The above established evidence provides a rationale for the use of DMT with children and adolescents. Despite the lack of research, the documentation supports the possibility that DMT may provide for a reduction in anxiety and an increase in expressiveness and verbal ability for populations such as the young offender (delinquent), E.B.D., learning disabled, and autistic, particularly where a favourable attitude to movement is present.

The available literature shows that DMT has been successfully practised with these populations and gives weight to its use in special schools where many of these children and adolescents are found.

Psychotherapy

DMT has links with psychotherapeutic theory. Definitions of psychotherapy vary from the relief of neurosis to the art of relieving psychiatric problems by psychological means. It is often referred to as 'verbal therapy' or simply 'therapy'. The many varieties of psychotherapy have different theoretical frameworks. Some pursue the task of understanding by using the concepts of the patient, others reconstruct the meaning within some new language. All seek the best reading of the patient's material, that which captures most succinctly what they wish to communicate.

The goal of psychotherapy could be described as freeing the individual's ability to choose what they engage with and following through with them to 'bring about a reconciliation between the individual's feeling and social norms without sacrificing the integrity of the individual' (Watts 1973: 16).

From the literature, it would seem that counselling is more prevalent in schools than is psychotherapy (for example, Rabiochow and Sklansky 1980) and research shows it should be available in all secondary schools (Curtis and Gilmore 1982). It is of a one-to-one nature and is traditionally seen as part of the teacher's 'pastoral role' in the school. Special schools and community homes with education on the premises have psychologists and social workers who practise counselling, training in assertiveness skills, and stress release. Counselling has been used in the form of educational therapy to some effect with poor readers, with behaviour difficulties, and with those with learning difficulties. Most research in school settings (for example, Barcai et al. 1973) states that the therapist's personality, expectation, and attitudes are not enough to improve outcome. However, Kolvin et al. (1981), in an extensive UK research study, indicate that a therapist's assertiveness, openness, and extraversion are more relevant in the school setting with its fairly busy atmosphere. The sensitive, empathic therapist may be overwhelmed in a school which is not designed primarily for therapy. Research findings, which were not in a school setting, claim 'empathy, warmth and genuineness are the prerequisite qualities for good outcome' (Truax and Carkuff 1967: 73). Perhaps this indicates a need for the therapist to cultivate all these qualities. Nicol and Parker (1981) researched non-directive play group therapy in a junior school with encouraging results; however, De Martino (1986) analysed several school-based psychotherapy studies and showed it to be only moderately effective.

Research in psychotherapy for young people in clinical settings is normally concerned with family, behavioural, group, and individual therapy with severely disturbed adolescents; few studies are on the use of body/mind therapies. The young people are not labelled as having 'learning difficulty' or being 'delinquent' although in essence they may be. Rutter and Giller (1982) suggest that behaviour change using psychotherapy and intensive counselling may be possible with a minority of delinquents who are highly anxious and want help. It may be concluded that an adolescent with a neurotic or anxiety score in an assessment test is more likely to have a disturbance associated with their delinquency than one with a nil score. This minority is more likely to respond positively to a therapeutic process, especially one that is largely non-verbal and essentially active.

The use of groups in the psychiatric setting is prevalent and such treatment the norm. However, despite all the curriculum opportunities taking place in groups in schools, there is a reluctance to embrace group therapy, even where the population is troubled or troublesome, unless it is in a private school such as Bridgeways (1985), usually called a therapeutic community. Research is very scant.

It is therefore more important to make a case for these children and adolescents to benefit from the services offered by the therapies in the school setting than in the psychiatric setting where such work is seen as highly relevant and DMT may be more easily adapted for use.

Research results tend to favour behavioural as opposed to play or verbal therapy, but this could be due to behavioural therapy dealing with overt 'symptoms' and desensitization, and the ease with which outcome studies can be applied. Many of the studies are school-based, some from psychiatric samples, including residential homes for delinquents and disruptive underachieving or behaviour problem boys.

In summary, although educational theory, practice, and experience influenced early pioneers in the field of group therapy (many were teachers initially) there has been little application in the school system to date. However, creative activities and play in a supportive, democratic, socially aware atmosphere are significant in the literature. The reason for the educational emphasis may be that schools are where children and adolescents are usually located and where most of their behaviours are manifested. Counselling programmes, rather than psychotherapy, are present in schools (mainstream and special); it may be that a counselling function is an appropriate home base for DMT.

An approach such as DMT, with structures where the child or adolescent can explore what they can 'do' in action may be a useful midway approach between the totally client-centred, verbal and environmental treatments.

Infant and adolescent development

When we are working with these groups it is important to recognize that the relationship between mother and infant provides the necessary conditions for healthy ego development. The mother's nurturing enables a merging to occur where she empathizes with the infant and keeps a space for its needs, giving meaning to the chaos which the infant cannot yet give. These repeated experiences of having a space in someone's mind and of being understood enable the infant to develop its own capacity to think. This process is reflected physically in the holding of the infant by the mother, the space given by her bodily creation of a 'container'.

The fulfilment of needs gives a sense of omnipotence and well-being. However, the mother can never fulfil all the needs, so frustrations are experienced by the infant, particularly at times of separation. Defence mechanisms develop to protect the infant from experiencing helplessness when letting go of mother. For the stage of separation to emerge mother also needs to let go of the infant. Loss is experienced in order to enter the next stage in relationship. Identity is established by the mother's ability to mirror and reflect back (Stern 1974; Lacan 1977) the infant's feelings as she understands them (Pines 1982). To come out of the fusion the infant needs to be able to hold an image of mother whilst she is absent. The senses of self as identified by Stern (1985), once formed, function throughout life.

The above description is of the infant's postulated pre-verbal self-experience. This is the non-verbal, global, experiential knowledge about how inanimate things work, how their bodies work, and how social interactions work, before they are assembled into a verbal code. This pre-verbal domain is one of the most important aspects that can be addressed through DMT.

Many of the young people in special education make sense of their world from numerous negative life experiences. This leaves them less trusting and less open to the meaning of a particular situation. Since they are less open to the world their range of meaning is narrower. Eventually, only negative affective meaning is attributed by them; their meanings become less accessible to others, causing conflict.

Language is a powerful tool in communication, but the rich texture of a child's experience is difficult to express in speech. By using creative dance and movement as a therapeutic intervention, some of the limitations of speech do not apply and children often find ways to express ideas and feeling in metaphor or by symbol. In groupwork these can be felt and experienced by others. DMT is also appropriate for children with language, communication, or learning difficulties. They often enjoy moving up to an older age and so are less resistant to DMT than some mainstream children.

Anna Freud (1958) postulated that in adolescence sexual desires spark a resurgence of oedipal conflicts for boys. The importance of physical changes, peer groups, role models, parents, formation of identity, and the influence of the environment all need to be borne in mind. It is a time of turmoil that involves rapidly changing social, psychological, and physiological aspects. In the psychoanalytical model it is claimed that the upsurge of sexual and aggressive drives conflicts with identity, and difficulties with establishing sexual identity predominate for both boys and girls.

In the mid-teens physiological changes stabilize prior to the intra-psychic processes where the id, psychoanalytical material claims, shifts in favour of the ego. There is a major shift in love interest, where parental closeness is given up and boys and girls are attracted to each other. Abstract thinking abilities allow for instinctive drives to be dealt with in fantasy and thought rather than by impulsive action or excessive inhibition. The older male adolescent is more amenable to reason and is not so frightened of his sexual and aggressive drives. He may be more willing to co-operate and understand himself, for example in verbal psychotherapy. Both phases have recurrent alternations between disturbed behaviour and quiescence.

Features of the adolescent process as commonly described in psycho-analytic literature are: confusion, concern with painful separation, intense feelings manifested in adults, and problems encountered in applying the usual treatment procedures to those in difficulties during the adolescent process. Psychoanalytic theory is not, in fact, a sufficient theory of human behaviour, normal or abnormal. However, the ideas on dependency, repression, transference, and resistance are particularly useful. The humanistic or growth model and behaviourist system need to be considered, since they too offer useful guidelines for working with young people. The humanistic model is useful since it describes a positive view of growth which the author supports. This links to the behaviouristic view where learning can enable adolescents to satisfy some of their needs and resolve some of their conflicts, for example in learning assertion techniques.

Adolescence and delinquency

This subsection will enable the reader to understand the theoretical concepts underpinning the case illustration.

Many children and adolescents with a learning difficulty and/or emotional disturbance/conduct disorder also become offenders, particularly boys. There is also evidence that those of normal learning ability can be labelled delinquent. Typically conduct disordered offenders have exaggerated difficulties relating to authority figures which can be interpreted as negative transference. There is normally a poor self-concept which is influenced by social factors such as the attitudes of others, and that self-concept is usually reflected in the individual's attitudes towards others. Adolescent behaviour is a reflection of interaction between the individual and the environment. If delinquent, the adolescent separates from and de-idealizes parents and invests in friends and peer culture which may become manifest through gangs, glue sniffing, drugs, alcohol, sexual experimentation, or TV violence. However, like most adolescents, they identify with the pop music and disco dance culture which is helpful in enabling a movement attitude in DMT sessions, particularly when they are encouraged to bring their own music.

Psychoanalytic thought claims that delinquent behaviours derive from insoluble intrapsychic conflicts in the unconscious and that, through various combinations of inner and outer stresses and precipitating events, previously used methods of maintaining the equilibrium fail and symptoms or traits appear. In the patterning of these symptoms and associated character traits, which reveal elements of the inner conflicts, the ego's coping mechanisms can be seen. The aggressive impulses identified in the latency period (unruliness, naughtiness) thus become criminal behaviours. DMT, as the intervention used, is an action approach that may enable anxiety to be reduced. For some adolescents, though, action may not reduce anxiety but can act as an avoidance tactic, an alternative to confronting and resolving underlying conflicts. It is claimed that such repetitious action as delinquent behaviour is an acting out of unconscious conflicts symptomatic of a serious impediment to maturation.

Winnicott (1971) suggests that adolescents need to be given reality by an act of confrontation, which needs to be personal and containing and may be painful to execute. The power struggle is about the adult's removal and replacement. Winnicott would say this was tantamount to murder, that is, the destruction of the parents. The adolescent needs them to survive though; if they do not he feels let down. Bruce (1975) uses the concept of mirroring as a form of confrontation, reflecting back what is given by the adolescent. In DMT the technique of the therapist mirroring the client's movement material is sometimes useful with adolescents, creating a feedback loop whereby they can see something of themselves.

According to the humanistic model, when the individual lacks sufficient self-confidence to chart their course of actions openly, seems content to grow in self-realization vicariously rather than directly, and does little to channel this drive in constructive directions, then the individual is also said to be E.B.D. A barrier is reached and the individual cannot access self-realization, which results in resistance and friction. From the author's understanding, the drive towards self-realization is continual and the individual's behaviour demonstrates either that they have satisfied their inner drive by outwardly fighting to establish a self-concept in the world of reality, or that they have satisfied it vicariously by confusing it with their inner world. In the humanistic view, people's feelings of security and satisfaction depend on a sense of being able to exert control over the reactions of others towards them as well as over their own inner states.

The behaviourist theory of the process of development implies that all behaviour is learned through a set of stimuli and responses, reinforcement and extinction. Society controls behaviour so, this theory claims, adolescent behaviours are learned according to those stimuli and reinforcements available in the young person's environment. This assumes that conflicts, life-style, stress, hopes, and fears in adolescence are all learned and can be 'unlearned'. Eisler and Frederikson (1980) claim that social skills are largely responsible for life's development and are frequently used with adolescents. In my DMT practice, exploring ways of, for example, saying 'no' non-verbally enabled one young person to engage with the difficulties he experienced when attempting to stay out of trouble. His understanding of a dilemma he faced increased when, on returning to his home environment after a period of confinement, friends who were frequently 'in trouble with the law' would encourage him to join with them. He feared isolation and rejection if he did not participate, yet wished to remain 'clean' as during his incarceration.

II ONSTAGE

This section presents an account of some techniques, core concepts, and therapeutic strategies which have been found helpful when applying DMT as an intervention in special schools. The section concludes with a case illustrating a young offender's perceptions of the DMT process together with a discussion.

TECHNIQUES

The practice of DMT in special education

Since there are firm moves towards the recognition of DMT in the health service and only tentative beginnings for such recognition in education,[2] I should like to focus on arguing for its implementation in special education.

In the special school settings it was to my advantage that I am a qualified teacher and had gained further advanced training in special educational needs. I had previous experience of working with adolescents as a PE specialist in mainstream secondary education and therefore knew of the challenge. In both the school for moderate learning difficulties and later in a department for non-communicating children I was employed as a full-time staff member in a teacher's post which gave me the same conditions of service as teachers. There was ambivalence about my role since I was expected to offer movement and games lessons, do break duties, and take on a supervisory role for nursery nurses applying teaching strategies. However, generally there was a respect for my role as dance movement therapist, where time was negotiated for writing session notes and for supervision. Further information about the children was gained through the additional roles and was a baseline for their responses in the sessions. There were difficulties with the roles, particularly when interacting with those children in DMT sessions; outside the sessions, expectations might have been different. On reflection, these tensions increased my awareness of my values and approach in DMT. The children learned that the DMT sessions were different and special, unique in their atmosphere, distinct from movement lessons and play times. They could also appreciate that our DMT relationship began and ended with the session. Indirect observation of future referrals was possible and liaison with teachers and assistants was deeper. They were more able to trust me, I felt, as a conscientious member of the multi-disciplinary team. There was the problem of handling curious other children who wanted to come to sessions or asked about their content. Where my work was of a part-time nature there were fewer difficulties with clarification of role although the shortage of time made liaison more complex.

Several sessions were offered to staff in these settings to help them understand the differing roles of therapist and teacher. Invited speakers were employed to support this education process and give me some further input. This promoted staff support for the DMT opportunities and an increasing awareness about referrals, which in the early days had been for reasons such as lack of co-ordination, perceptual-motor difficulties, or physical handicap. Later referrals were for isolation, truancy, disruptive behaviour, and other reasons, although at times DMT sessions were also used by teachers to reward or punish, which was not helpful.

There needs to be a comment here on the differing roles and aims of DMT and teaching. For example, in teaching the focus is on specific learning outcomes whereas in therapy it is on inward processes. The contract is different in therapy where achievement is not seen to be the way to improve self-esteem. Part of the process is the transference of negative and positive feelings onto the therapist (stemming from early relationships); counter-transference is also acknowledged. Therapy is helpful where the child cannot form a trusting relationship with the teacher and where learning opportunities are not available because of emotional conflicts and learning problems. Skills are not normally taught in DMT, and therapists need to ensure they are not directed towards such goals. It would be helpful if dance education and special education teachers' courses included an understanding of DMT to help avoid fears and misunderstandings when DMT is practised in education. The training for teachers is different from the training in DMT. Teachers wishing to work in DMT would need to take a further postgraduate course to become dance movement therapists (see Appendix for details of training). Supervision is essential and personal therapy recommended since there is a need for the therapist to be aware of their own active part in the DMT processes (for elaboration on this issue, see Payne 1990).

Prior to 1988 there was no validated DMT training so dance and movement educators turned to dance and special education as the nearest model. As teaching has changed from a child-centred approach the role of DMT has become clearer. DMT can make a contribution similar to, yet different from, psychotherapy or counselling. It can complement the dance and movement teaching role which relates to movement skill, movement range, technique, and the making, presenting, performance, and criticism of dance. This process pays no attention to psychological development or the unconscious mind, although with the national curriculum, the personal and social areas[3] could overlap with some of the aims of DMT, particularly in special schools where the teacher–pupil relationship is regarded as more important. In any event, it is essential that the school acknowledges that DMT is the intervention offered and that staff selecting for referral know the processes it entails. There may be some envy from teachers, especially if the DMT sessions are one-to-one or in small groups, hence the importance of liaising with them by giving regular feedback to help their understanding and to promote a greater understanding of the child.

The dance movement therapist needs to be firm about what she and the sessions are called; for example, the terms 'teacher' and 'lesson' can lead to confusion and certain expectations from the children and staff. The child or adolescent often tries to make the therapist into a teacher, expressing, for example, a need to learn to dance or move more effectively; the therapist will need to be careful not to become drawn into praising or criticizing. In conclusion, introducing the practice of DMT in special schools has its difficulties, particularly over roles, although no more so I imagine than for a social worker or nurse with a DMT practitioner qualification. But there are some advantages over working in, for example, the health service where the salaries are pitifully low.

Core concepts

Here I will focus on two of the recurring core concepts with these populations, those of resistance and rejection. The material shows how these concepts are often manifested in the way these populations express themselves in DMT sessions. Extracts from my session notes help to illustrate the material. Following this and the introduction to therapeutic strategies, the case illustration is taken from a formal research project where the client's perceptions of the DMT process were documented and analysed.

Resistance

Graafsme and Anbeck describe resistance as

> behaviour that a person carries out in order to forestall the appearance of an unwelcome impulse, an affect or an action by himself or another. A resistance is a defensive response to sensation that threatens everyday functioning and the integration of internal and external stimuli.
>
> (Graafsme and Anbeck 1984: 3)

Graafsme and Anbeck found that adolescents were curious about psychotherapy at first, the unknown being alluring but frightening. However, they are often curious about unusual or interesting activities. There does seem to be a general resistance to painful feelings in all groups; adolescents in particular also fear influences which may render them helpless and ashamed. Receiving help may be interpreted by them as acknowledging failure and, in the author's experience of disordered adolescents, it is almost impossible for them to recognize that they need help.

The traditional analytical approach to resistance has been interpretation; that is, verbal acknowledgement to the young person. Adelman and Taylor (1986) claim that adolescents' reluctance to participate in psychotherapy may be the result of their appropriate negative perceptions of the treatment. It is important to be aware of both possibilities, and there is no simple way of distinguishing between them.

The adolescent needs to retain their sense of 'active mastery' of their world. Fear of loss of control often leads to an extensive resistance to emotional investment in the therapist. Themes such as control versus loss of control or loyalty and dependency versus independence are usual. For example, in one DMT group for young offenders with high anxiety, each member was encouraged to become 'the controller', for 'The Talk Dance' game where they conducted the others through a sequence of movements from their own ideas to music. The therapist derived the theme from the previous sessions' material such as 'holding back in slow motion' or 'jumping away from the world'.

The presence of resistance expressed by a lack of motivation does not necessarily mean that the adolescent has no desire to change. The author believes that there is an implicit wish to take up healthy development again. The need to be accepted by and belong to society may be represented by a significant adult; the therapist therefore needs to be able to be idealized as a significant other in order for a working alliance to develop. This cannot take place if prevailing material is not recognized and worked through in the early stages. It is often the case that negative transference becomes the overriding process in the development of the group.

There are problems around the following issues which commonly arise in DMT practice with groups in educational settings as a manifestation of resistance: a) boredom, b) absence, c) physical contact.

a) Boredom

In contrast to the need for physical movement expressed by children and adolescents, this issue can also surface. Often, engagement can be maintained for only short periods of time; the excuses are often 'this is too boring', 'this is stupid', or 'I feel bloody daft doing this'. This can be understood in terms of resistance, a defence against change and a protection from exposure.

From my notes:

> G thought the Territory Dance was boring – we sat and stared at a spot on the mat to explore the boringness – others said this too was boring and that G was attention seeking again. I'm feeling very disillusioned after this session, the clients' own journals mostly said how boring the session was and that they nearly fell asleep!

b) Absence

Pretending to sleep is one way of being absent from the group and a common behavioural response when 'bored'. By accepting this 'sleeping' and waiting or working with the stillness the therapist conveys an understanding which enables a reawakening to action before long. Other apparent absenteeism is manifested through 'hiding' games, in cupboards or under chairs, for example. These are usefully engaged with, leading to 'seeking' behaviour and further experimentation, such as moving with eyes closed or blindfolded. These behaviours, often in the early stage of the group's life, may relate to the fear of being seen by the therapist.

Sometimes there is constant clock watching, requesting the time, or asking how much longer and so on, again a clear message of not wanting to be present with the therapist and the group. Most of the suggestions made by the therapist for movement are rejected at first, then later they are worked with for short bursts. However, there may be a struggle with the engagement for disturbed and conduct disordered groups as reflected in play fights, swearing, uncontrolled movement, and the throwing of objects.

From my notes with a group of young offenders:

> They had nothing in the space they could use as missiles so they began tearing up the plastic tiles and lobbing them at each other. It felt totally chaotic. Their ambivalence is clearly shown in their bold requests to each other to 'stop messing a'boot and get on with it' in contrast to their shouting that the movement is stupid and I am boring.

Occasionally young people will leave the space if it becomes too painful or frightening for them to remain. Others will simply not arrive at the session, claiming to have forgotten or be involved in another, more interesting project. If the session is at the same time as maths or another unpopular activity they will normally come to DMT willingly. Sometimes the young person will enlist the support of a parent to write to request they be excused because of a cold. Many times non-participation in DMT is manifested in a body-based problem: 'I have a pain' or 'My lunch is not digested' or 'I cannot move today, I hurt my leg', and so on. Part of the space can be given to those not wanting to move as an opportunity to be present whilst frequently being encouraged to join in.

From my notes:

> Comments from all except M who sat in the corner where S normally sits and said nothing. The theme of 'running away' was worked through somewhat by encouraging running through the space and asking what they might be running towards or from. Asking what else could they do with their legs if they did not run, some lay on backs and thrust legs about and banged on the floor in tantrum movements. One member chased the others but it seemed too much for them and a fight developed between chaser and one runner. I had to ask one boy to go for help to separate them. It's not worth all the hassle, I feel like giving up on them. Nothing is working, chaos always ensues. I felt helpless having to have help. Will I be seen as failing to control them, will I be respected by staff?

The latter part indicates I am doubting my capacity to be the container of the chaos.

c) Physical contact

One of the common difficulties with latency and adolescent-aged young people is the issue of touch, which is an integral aspect of DMT practice (Montague 1971; Willis 1987). Adolescents fear physical contact, particularly boys. They cannot cope with the therapist's touch, for example, if there is confusion between touch as a caring gesture and touch as intrusion in physical aggression or sexual violation. Touching is often regarded by them as being concerned with being gay, perverted, or aggressive.

Structures which include touch need to be carefully designed. The stress may be on not touching whilst shadow boxing in pairs, for example. Props which connect the group such as parachutes, stretchy material, or elastic can sometimes be safer for such groups. At other times the athleticism required by contact improvisation or balance work in small groups can include touch in a manner which is acceptable to them (Scott 1988).

Associated with touch is sexuality, a common issue amongst adolescents. Laufer and Laufer (1984) contend that the psychopathology of the severely disturbed adolescent has its source in conflicts over the sexually mature body, maintaining that some impairment exists in their capability to relate to their bodies in a caring way. Much of my work necessarily centred on self-massage, tension-reducing exercises, and a general caring for their bodies in an attempt to begin an awareness of self-care. The issue of sexuality becomes easily interwoven within the therapeutic alliance particularly when touch arises out of the dance in the group or in relaxation structures where, for example, the therapist might massage the client's shoulders or head:

> In touching the patient we very easily open up the possibility of preverbal transferences . . . we set up conditions whereby the patient may fuse with the therapist as an infant would. Intense dependency needs are often evoked which are not entirely in the patient's awareness. . . . Sometimes these early needs can appear to the patient as strong sexual attraction to the therapist.
>
> (McNeely 1987: 77)

From my notes with an all-male group:

> The structure of the participants each choosing a different name to represent their identity at that point and moving its qualities led to N acting effeminate and putting socks up his jumper for breasts. Others said their walks reflected 'gays', 'poofters', and 'a beating someone up walk'. All the things they most fear perhaps, all the

confusing thoughts concerned with their relationship with me as a female, identity, the macho and the feminine sides. . . . In the group today I felt M was touching me with a sensuality in our contact work, someone else said to a participant 'don't touch me I'm not gay' when we did falling and catching. . . . The boys' journals read 'J wants to make love with you, wants sex with you, he loves you', 'You have a bloody sexy body, I wouldn't mind getting my end away with you'. . . . It feels threatening and risky for me to work with them next week.

For some populations, such as those labelled delinquent, there is little opportunity to combine girls and boys since the settings mostly contain boys. With autistic and learning disabled children there is less of a problem and mixed groups are possible. However, in adolescent work there is often less involvement from girls if boys are present also. If girls' clothing is unsuitable for movement or floor work they complain, or simply do not turn up that day. Given the stages of sexual and social development, this is understandable. PE lessons are taken separately at this age for such reasons. However, single-sex groupings of all girls or all boys with a female therapist will, predictably, have an effect on the issues for those groups, as will a mixed grouping.

Rejection

Another important concept recurring in these populations is that of abandonment. In practice this is linked to being left, for example, when the therapist is absent through illness or holidays or in the final stages of therapy. The learning disabled and delinquent are often emotionally disturbed in addition; no one knows which preceded which. Some are from stable homes but many are not. Research studies indicate that deprivation in early life may have serious effects on the child's capacity to establish trusting and secure relationships as well as on the ability to think and learn (Ainsworth 1962; Britton 1978; Bowlby 1951, 1979; Holmes 1980). Holmes (1983) highlights early deprivation leading to learning difficulties being recurrent enough to suggest a link between deprivation and the capacity to retain knowledge and think. Thinking is related to emotional development, the space in the mind to receive the mental equivalent of food evolved from the mother's capacity to contain the chaos of painful feelings and sensations emanating from the infant and her own ability to give meaning to the meaningless. Autistic, psychotic, or profoundly handicapped children have normally been diagnosed when infants or young children. It is unclear how the unusual pattern of withdrawal from the mother, and the world, arises, for example, whether it was first initiated by the child, in response to its confused inner world or to the parent, or whether the parent, upset and rejecting of her handicapped child, made the move which led to a cycle of rejection on both sides. The delinquent adolescent has normally experienced a disrupted home life and presents as 'difficult' to get close to. The rejection felt is often experienced as physical abandonment, which, if it cannot be undone by finding a sexual partner, could lead to psychosomatic expression of depressed feelings.

Thus many children and adolescents in these groups experienced frequent changes in their short lives, having been in several schools, foster homes, assessment centres, hospital and care facilities. They were often emotionally deprived, some severely disturbed, often having experienced many rejections, particularly from parental figures. Parents would have similarly experienced a breakdown of their home environment through divorce or abandonment and frequently been received into care themselves.

From my notes:

> During the second half of the session we worked with giving weight to each other, sharing weight on backs. They were sensitive to each other, necks very tense. . . . I encouraged a 'giving' of themselves to their partner. A theme arose during the talking period of 'being thrown away'. They asked if I had ever given anybody away – I replied no, they continued questioning – are you married? Will you have kids? Will you give any of your kids away? G said his mum had given him away, he still loves her though, his foster family is OK but not the same. I said it must hurt, 'Yes, it does' he replied chokingly. 'They can't handle us that's why they give us away' said P. Now I feel we are getting to the heart of some important issues for them. Feelings emerged today concerned with longing, love, anger, sadness and hurt. . . . It was a sad session for me, really depressed at their past and current lives.

Any lack of containment or bonding experienced by the mother as a child may disable her when empathizing with her infant. She may feel overwhelmed by the connection with her own early fears. She may feel the child's anxiety as persecutory; there is a cycle of demands which results in rejection as they cannot be met.

Children who have been emotionally deprived and who have experienced rejection, such as many of the learning disabled and delinquent populations, are likely to have lacked early experiences of 'good enough' mothering and they will have developed defences against dependence and overwhelming anxiety. They feel safest with structured, repetitive tasks but are often unable to concentrate for long on even these.

Some groups will enact the fury of being shut out and left unloved, and their resentment and hate are difficult for those staff seen as parental figures who try to make a relationship. They unconsciously aim to make the adult repeat the response that is known and familiar, confirming their self-image as 'bad'. The result is that they are again rejected by the staff or school as being too difficult or inappropriately placed.

Boys will often respond differently from girls to their deprivation. They are more defensive, as manifested in their body armouring, muscular and rigid, and have an air of bravado, aiming to keep unemotional. A therapist's opposite gender can bring out issues of rejection of all things female, and if the word 'dance' is used it sometimes compounds their flight from the work. The outpouring of aggression helps in their denial of the underlying sadness. Where there is a 'secure order' or a residential placement, issues of hostility are often directed at the school itself and absconding is frequent.

From a research volunteer's journal (journals were individually completed prior to the end of each group session. The therapist read them and made an entry prior to the following session, a kind of private message system): 'I wanted to stamp on your [the therapist's] hand because I am a bastard and I wanted to hurt you . . .'.

Table 3.1 gives an overview of some DMT approaches suggested when working with resistance/rejection for one particular grouping.

Table 3.1 Common issues, core concepts, and suggested approaches in DMT groupwork with delinquent and disturbed adolescents

Issues	Concepts	Approach
Boredom	Resistance	Stimulate through varying pace and tasks in early stages, e.g. competitive movement games and self-competition.
Absence, lethargy	Resistance	Non-action, nurturing structures where the fear of being 'seen' by therapist is theme.
High anxiety	Resistance	Relaxation exercises or discharge of energy through vigorous movement. Clear ground rules.
Dependency/sexuality	Rejection	Clear boundaries. Playful action
Fear of self-disclosure	Rejection	No pressure, keep in abstract, not relating to real life.
Authority issues	Resistance and rejection	Therapist low profile, group analytic dance approach, group as focus.
Self-consciousness (fear of touch)	Rejection	All move at the same time, e.g. theme – we are all looked at by each other.
Fear of exclusion	Rejection	Each take a turn, we are all looked at individually by each other.

Therapeutic strategies

There are a number of strategies which are important to employ when working with children and adolescents. Several are outlined here to give the reader a sense of the way practice could proceed with these groups. Methods such as *joining*, and the idea of the *moving therapist* are discussed, together with underlining the importance of *space*, the implementation of *ground rules*, coping with the young person's *withdrawal from class* for sessions, and the use of *combined treatment approaches* and *assessment and evaluation*.

Joining

Identified by Marshall (1982) as 'joining', the child is actively joined by the therapist in a variety of ways. Moving with the child has been a well-established technique in DMT, the therapist reflecting the child's movement by shadowing, echoing, mirroring, and so on. Another approach is to give a running commentary on whatever is happening in the movement. Its starting point lies in the movement created by the child. By verbalizing the movement, it takes on a special meaning. For example, Jane had stopped discussing her feelings of hurt by her peers at school and begun to move her hands: 'You are moving your fingers out and in; now you are pressing them into each other hard.'

There is no attempt at interpretation of the child's feelings or thoughts but an active focus on the movement material presented. The verbalization needs to be reflective of the quality of the movement in its tone and pace. It needs to convey an implicit acceptance of whatever is going on yet give form to the movement action and interaction, promoting an extension. This type of commentary translates the movement content, feelings, and meanings into a structure and encourages participation from the child. Often they begin to talk about what they are doing and so further communication emerges. For those children with chaotic thinking and acting it furthers differentiation of experiences and information processing. Sounds may clarify the meaning of the movement, for example accenting the breath or adding stamps, groans, sighs, and all manner of expressive vocalizations. Sometimes the use of percussion is helpful.

Children are not obliged to acknowledge openly that their personal difficulties, thoughts, and feelings are being worked with. They can stay hidden in the safe symbol or metaphor of the movement.

Many children do not have access to their creative movement potential and may need stimuli to begin. By suggesting possible ways of starting and by modelling movement activity they normally respond. With children who have learning difficulties it is often more helpful if the therapist is direct in suggesting movement ideas throughout the session.

For some, using developmental movement stages such as the early motor activity of grasp and release may be useful depending upon the child's level of functioning.

The moving therapist

Since the therapist's role is often active and with the client, in the movement she is able to:

a) influence the form and content of the movement in the direction of the therapeutic aims and objectives;
b) model the many possibilities in movement;
c) open a path to communication at a pre-verbal level;
d) engage the client in movement by showing that movement is desirable and important.

Her intervention influences both the expression of the experience and the experience itself and therefore themes arise and are selected in relation to therapeutic aims and objectives. The range of movement the therapist possesses will influence the movement interaction as will the feelings the therapist has about their body and movement, in general and in the presence of the particular group.

Space

It is important to have a consistent space for DMT sessions, one which is not used for regular lessons or other activities. Associations with spaces can make the work more difficult; for example, a space used with an adolescent group was also a 'holding room' at break times. The comics and crisp packets were the least of the problem because the young people had got used to lying on the cupboards, fighting, and so on. Distractions such as mobiles need to be removed as do desks and chairs. If possible, a space which is away from the main corridor is advisable since privacy is essential; curious others often seem to find the sessions more interesting than the group! Any windows in walls or doors need to be covered and a sign on the door may help restrain interruptions from both staff and pupils.

Ground rules

Firm boundaries are essential, particularly with adolescents. The times of sessions need to be adhered to by the therapist and the young people informed of them well in advance. It is not advisable to change the time or day of sessions. Often this is a difficulty when schools arrange trips, or parents or social workers visit.

There will normally need to be rules with sanctions within the context of the session to enable the young person to feel secure; usually these need to be agreed by everyone. For example, no physical violence against self, others, or equipment; arriving on time; staying in the space; no smoking; commitment to sessions; and confidentiality. In one group there was a decision to have a 'no swearing' rule with ten press-ups for any offenders. I have only once used exclusion from the group as a sanction and that was for violence.

Withdrawal from the classroom

Although many children will be withdrawn for various reasons such as individual remedial lessons, speech therapy, physiotherapy, and so on, the DMT session is special because it is the one time they can creatively explore their conflicts and fears in a contained setting. Lessons often set up more conflict for such children and withdrawal gives a sense of relief and provides for the need for attention.

The times of return need to mesh with breaks, lunch, or the end of lessons in order to give the children an opportunity to merge easily back into the school. There can be difficulties when collecting younger or less able children or adolescents who may feel embarrassed about leaving peers. Other pupils or the teacher may make an unhelpful remark. Some are able to come to sessions alone.

A group session can easily be timed to fit into a lesson of forty minutes, whereas individual slots of fifteen to thirty minutes are more difficult to arrange without the withdrawal and return of the child to the classroom.

Combined approaches

This refers to combined individual and group DMT sessions with the same therapist. From research into combined group and individual therapy programmes, it seems the group experience brings out problems of adjustment not possible in individual sessions. The latter focus more sharply on the individual, providing for trust and security and eliminating the stimulus for activity received in the group situation.

Pfeifer and Spinner (1985) recommend combined individual and group psychotherapy with children, preferably with the same therapist for both. Reasons are varied, including that the same therapist provides for a wider view of the child, a stronger alliance with the child, and a broader treatment approach, which, it is claimed, is most effective with the child most resistant yet most in need of treatment.

Slaveson and Schiffer (1975) theorize that the child suffering from severe parental deprivation cannot be treated exclusively in activity group therapy. Anna Freud (1965) noted that children do not form negative transference neuroses *per se* but rather relate to the therapy in a manner she termed 'substitutive'; that is, they generally do not enter treatment motivated to form a therapeutic alliance. She recommends the use of individual therapy to gratify the child and the group to confront maladaptive behaviours and defences.

On the basis of assessment information a judgement is then made as to whether the child is suitable for DMT and, if so, whether an individual, dyad, group, or combined approach is best. The length, review stages, and type of programme are decided; for example, it may be more conducive to keep children, latency ages, and adolescents in separate groups since their developmental needs are different. Integrated groups have been found to be possible, for example, those with moderate learning difficulties and autistic children.

Assessment and evaluation

DMT is only effective if a thorough assessment is made of the child or adolescent and, where applicable, the family's problems. Upon referral there is a need a) to identify whether DMT is specifically required; b) to define the overall aims and objectives for the programme; and c) to determine what strategies or techniques might be most effective. Movement observation can give important information particularly where individual work is anticipated.

When the staff are given an understanding of the processes of DMT, referrals become more appropriate. After referral the child needs to be assessed with the help of, for example, psychological tools and movement observation. Consultation with teachers, parents, and social workers follows, together with an interview with the child to find out further information such as how they perceive their problems, to explain the idea of DMT, and possibly to set goals together for the DMT sessions.

In my practice, anxiety ratings, social adjustment guides, ьnd other forms of psychological assessment procedure have been useful in the selection of groups for DMT. For example, it was found that to mix those identified as 'withdrawn' with 'inconsequential' or 'hostile' people as defined by Stott's Social Adjustment Guide led to difficulties in group cohesion. For another adolescent group the young people completed an anxiety scale (Spielberger 1983) and identified their own goals for sessions based on their score results. For the most part selection for DMT has been on the basis of high anxiety, depression, or behavioural disturbance, and therapeutic aims and objectives set in consultation with staff and after reading case files.

With some anxious children and adolescents pre-treatment interviews only heighten the anxiety and can result in stronger resistance to sessions and with others they may be unsuitable because of communication difficulties. A demonstration session may serve diagnostic purposes also. Session evaluations need to include the pre-plan and final action involved, individuals' responses, the group's responses to the therapist and vice versa, group dynamics, movement material themes initiated by clients or therapist, and future objectives. In addition, a recording of the therapist's own experience is essential in order to differentiate the counter-transference and transference issues arising which may be addressed in supervision, and, if necessary, worked through in personal therapy. Both formative and summative evaluations need to relate to the therapeutic aims and objectives.

CASE ILLUSTRATION

This is the case of a young person who participated in a formal research project which explored the client's perceptions of a DMT group process with the author (Payne 1986, 1987, 1988a, 1988b). For the purpose of this chapter he is called Steve. Much of the text is his sense-making of the process. However, I then make an analysis of his perceptions, drawing together details from his file, staff comment, and my own understanding of childhood and adolescent development within this population. The slow building of the therapeutic relationship, work with parents and colleagues, assessment and objectives setting, and many of the decisions made during the sessions are omitted. Please keep in mind that more happened than can be shared here, but I have retained those aspects I believe to be important. Steve participated in individual sessions at first, followed by a few dyad sessions before entering one of two DMT groups for eight months. Confidentiality has been maintained through change of name and disguise of some details. Permission for the research and its documentation was given by adolescents, parents, and the school.

Steve, 14 years

Steve was a slim, lithe, good-looking boy of average height. He had dark-brown hair and a somewhat scruffy appearance. He was placed on a residential supervision order in a residential special school for those 'in care' because of persistent truancy, being out of parental control, and offences including assault to an elderly lady with the intention of robbing her. At risk in the community, he was suffering from some level of emotional disturbance having became stuck emotionally at a young age, when his parents separated five years previously when he was 8 years of age. He does see his father but cannot tolerate his new one (the mother's live-in boyfriend). Seen as a bully by boys and staff, he is able to show grief and anger but expresses rage with physical violence and spitting. He follows a remedial education programme.

His movement is well co-ordinated and fluctuates from free to bound flow and quick vibrancy to lethargy. He rarely makes eye contact, his chin being dropped onto his chest when he is talking. Most times he is very quiet, not paying attention and rarely initiating contact, seemingly quite tense.

Overall therapeutic aims of DMT group:

1 To work 'with' and 'against' another.
2 To work in threes, fours, and with the therapist individually in the group, taking turns to observe.
3 To disclose observations of self and others.
4 To work with objects such as percussion as an accompaniment.
5 To develop risk-taking.
6 To work with the issue of exclusion.

Extracts from therapist's case notes

Steve was a member of Group Two together with G, T, and R. The group ran for twenty-eight sessions, once a week. It took place in a small gymnasium which had a curtained stage in front of which hung some gym ropes.

There are several issues which emerged for Steve. His anger was noticeable. He commented several times on anger, particularly as expressed in physical aggression. I am aware he trod on people and crashed into them, mainly the weaker members of the group such as T. The other young people indicated similar perceptions. His file refers to several violent displays where he had both expressed and threatened physical damage to others. His comments included: 'when she falls it's funny', referring to me in one session with enjoyment at the possibility of my being hurt; 'I never let them stop – they were knackered', relating to when he was playing the drums for a 'chase me/catch me' improvisation and seemed to enjoy wearing the other boys out completely; 'I stood on his fingers 'cos I didn't see them'; 'if others say it too much I bop them', referring to taunts of other boys outside sessions regarding his participation as cissy; and 'I felt angry – I'll kick him in the balls', referring to a teacher who refused to allow him to come to his session one time as a punishment. Steve expressed extreme hostility and verbally abused the teacher considerably. The teacher had let T go to the session but not Steve, so possibly this was an expression of envy. He had four brothers, the elder and younger of whom received most of their mother's attention. He had taken to refusing to wash himself, perhaps as another method of drawing attention to the mother's apparent neglect of him.

His file's report of his punching, kicking, tripping behaviours were supported by other group members' comments heard outside the sessions: 'I was standing up 'cos I couldn't bend 'cos Steve had his feet out so I chickened out on that bit, I didn't want to because he was kicking me in the guts'. Here the group member was probably referring to an incident on the ropes when T left the session – this may well have been accidental. 'Steve batters and punches me' was another similar comment. I had also noticed how Steve intentionally tried to hurt my foot with a wooden plank in an individual session. This may have related to his anger at the imminent closing of the programme, which he could have been displaying towards me. He did enjoy the sessions and expressed desires for the next one to 'hurry up and arrive' even though his final comment at the end was a denial of this – 'they were just something that happened'. Another comment from my notes indicates my concern at his hurtful attitude to others: 'I had to explain the rules again about no hurting of self, others and property, S squeezed T's hand and hurt him', and 'S frequently let go suddenly when we were all in a group, wrists to wrists in contact, leaning out, or physically tried to destroy any cohesiveness'. This was early in the programme. Possibly he needed to sabotage any group contact to begin with in order to symbolize his own isolation and inadequate family grouping. His file stated that his parents were separated and that he could not accept his mother's new partner, wanting her to choose him, according to the psychiatrist's viewpoint, so causing animosity between himself and his mother. He was seen to be full of anger and found opportunities through bullying to express this. The sessions were no exception although, as one boy commented, 'he only bullies outside, not inside the sessions' which may indicate they felt he was less of a bully in DMT. As time went on he seemed to be more controlled within the sessions, although there was sabotaging the group physically, as in the group-lean which required physical contact and sharing of weight, and the opportunity to manipulate a movement interaction into a hurtful experience of another, reflecting his own hurt perhaps. His file notes he refused to care for his own body; perhaps this reflects parental neglect in infancy, perhaps he has been physically hurt in the past. He was less disruptive and demanding towards the end of the sessions, in particular there was less physical hurting of others, indicating a more caring attitude perhaps.

How did Steve make sense of the group? The research approach used methods of interview and journal writing to collect the client's experience of the DMT process. What follows is my sense-making of Steve's comments from this data.

Steve commented frequently on the group and the individuals in it. Outside the DMT sessions he mentioned those activities where they had worked as a group and made clear statements about interactions between group members in structures and improvisations. For example, 'we were boarding [clinging onto] each other, it was good, working with them, I liked them doing that', referred to a developing theme in the group which culminated in swinging on a rope with music as the accompaniment. On the beat, each in turn leapt and held the same rope so that all four were in contact and swinging before all dropped as a group onto the crash mat, often with much laughter. He referred to the activity as 'work', which may indicate his motivation and involvement despite viewing it as somewhat serious. It did require judgement, courage, physical contact with others, fitness, strength, timing, and sensitivity to others as well as play: 'everybody does the same movement', 'it's good working with them because it gives me a good feeling'. He may have enjoyed the synchrony of the whole group swinging at the same time; perhaps it gave him a feeling of 'togetherness', which possibly was rare in his family and experience since he seemed distanced from his peers. Swinging is a tension building to tension releasing activity, it is comforting like rocking. The activity on the ropes consisted of holding or clinging to the 'object' and letting go onto a safe floor.

At times his rivalry for attention was apparent. For example, he was able to give others attention whilst one member moved all over the space with the rest of the group, including him, accompanying on the drums; he particularly enjoyed playing and moving to the drum with strong, vital movements – an expression of his anger perhaps. He said this was good fun.

On one occasion about half-way through the programme R went up on the window ledge with a drum and wouldn't come down, so Steve climbed up too and played the drum. He said of this event, 'It was good up there with the sun shining in, making up my own music'. The theme emerging was moving up and away from the ground versus being low down on the floor under a parachute, or others who contributed passive weight. In this session Steve again used the drums as a way of expressing anger and as an accompaniment to R's daring circus act of swinging, hanging, and dropping. He then created his own climbing dance, ending up with the drum making music on the window ledge, so modelling R. However, he was able to rejoin the group easily. I decided not to make any intervention. Perhaps Steve saw this as a time for him to be alone and away from the intensity of the group interaction. Taking flight by being high up he could have been excluding himself, although not totally since we could hear his drumming most clearly, the noise somewhat excluding us! I bent over down on the ground with my hands on my ears. He had seen my intervention with R encouraging him to join us since there was possible danger, but Steve shut out my concern for him with his noisy drumming and I decided not to make any contact. He was clearly enacting the fury of being shut out and left unloved by a parental figure. I did feel helpless but decided not to reflect back his resentment (shout at him). Paradoxically he came down without any suggestion from me; perhaps he was more dependent than I thought; if he cannot gain my attention by being away from the group he will participate in the group for it. He seemed to see the sessions as a group interaction yet with the space to withdraw, if necessary. He saw my posture showing how he excluded me with his drumming and being so far away. Perhaps this reflected his reality of mother being angry with him resulting in her choosing a new man in his eyes, leaving Steve helpless and shut out. Clearly there was transformation in this moment of process and interaction.

His comment 'I was shy at first but not now because I can see how they [the other participants] react; I know them better now' seems perceptive. He was aware of other people's reactions and could use these as a means of 'knowing' them. Perhaps his withdrawal was a fear that they would reject him, destroy him, or let him destroy them with his anger. He stated that his shyness existed because he didn't know me or the others very well, adding 'it's our instinct to get shy'. Videotape recordings of sessions aided this self-perception (Furman 1990). He particularly commented on his shyness in relation to the video, saying that it startled him when he heard they would be videotaped and that he was shy at first that a stranger to the group would be coming in. Shyness, it seemed, was in reaction to 'unknown' people. He showed reflective ability, sensitivity, and awareness of his feelings in this disclosure to others.

In relation to me, Steve viewed me as a teacher, called me 'Miss' and seemed to have a positive attitude towards me. He told another adult that 'she is like any other teacher but a wee bit better', although he could not say what the better bit was when asked. My role with him, from his perception, was clearly not acknowledged as one of a therapist. This population's first response to offers of help, or any implication that they need another's assistance, is normally one of rejection. The term therapy is equated with sickness (or worse, madness, often their greatest fear) in their eyes. Other comments included 'she's a good teacher 'cos she lets you swing on the ropes and does some movements with you', indicating that teachers may not have allowed him to swing on the ropes, 'she joins in with you', 'she does what you do, copies you, plays follow my leader, all we do she does', 'she tries to do somersaults – not that good at it', which may all refer to my 'joining activities' where I moved in synchrony or echoed, mirrored, shadowed, and contrasted the essence of the group or individual's movement expression. He seemed to see me as having power I could use to deprive him; for example, he thought that I could say 'go back to class and don't come back' (although in fact this was not discussed as a sanction with this group), and that I had to set the ground rules. This relates to the core concept of rejection discussed earlier, where unconsciously the adolescent aims to make the adult repeat the response that is familiar, confirming them as 'bad' or 'not good enough' to participate. He was usually able to contribute something when we sat on mats and talked. Once when he was unable to finish an activity which he enjoyed due to lack of time he seemed very hurt when I reminded them of the time. He saw me as both depriving him yet also protecting him 'You hold the ropes back so they don't bump and hurt us' was a comment he made during our discussion about what we'd noticed about each other today. He had some ideas for improvement to sessions such as 'doing half dance, half talking and ten minutes swinging on the ropes; this', he said, 'is the fairest because you cannot do what we can do swinging on the ropes'. He saw this as giving me the opportunity for joining in some activities with them but that the rope activity was their special thing.

Comment

Steve perceived his gains as learning how to relax properly, how to move his body, getting a 'skive', and becoming fitter. He said that he would have to think about it before he would join a similar project.

From his perceptions and from cross-referencing to his file and other comments, it seems that the most prominent dimensions of Steve's experience of the sessions were concerned with 'his expression of anger' and 'participation in groupwork'. DMT may therefore have provided him with some way of expressing and acknowledging his anger in a safe way. He could symbolically destroy the group and express his wish to destroy me yet become one with the group within the structure of 'swinging together and release from the rope'. The 'falling forever' concept put forward by Winnicott (1962) refers to a child's anxiety when mother's care is not good enough. The group worked with falling (from the rope or in the form of jumping) for many weeks. The working through of this theme enabled the group to move on to work with anger and experiment further with participation.

DMT also facilitated group interaction in which he was able to experience a positive relationship through creative movement play and the forming of interactions which enhanced rather than invalidated his sense of self. Instead of feeling excluded (rejected) when not moving himself he was able to engage in observation and become, for example, the controller of other members' movement. There were times when he did exclude himself if things became too painful for him; however, by the therapist accepting and reflecting bodily his need for this and her non-directive intervention, he was able to rejoin the group. Disclosure of observations of self and the therapist were more frequent than those about others. As Steve became more trusting of the therapist and other group members 'seeing' him and accepting his painful feelings, his physical aggression in sessions lessened considerably, which enabled him to work creatively with others in movement structures. He absented himself from the group twice, and spent some time in sessions retreating from participation or engaging in 'hiding' behaviour. In the early sessions only when he was 'the controller' as in his drumming for others to move, for example, was he able to participate. His ambivalence was reflected in this way.

CONCLUSIONS

There have been many discoveries about the work over the time I practised in educational settings. However, I would like to share with you those conclusions about DMT and my understanding of the work which became evident in retrospect.

My personal therapy during this period played an important part in understanding DMT with these populations. I learned that children and adolescents were often very dependent on adults. Some probably always would be dependent to some extent, particularly the autistic and psychotic groups. The adolescents with labels such as 'delinquency' manifested themes which were necessarily about authority and power since this was their overriding experience. For example, one group worked with hiding, in their coats, under the mats, and in the cupboards. In supervision my own feelings about dealing with the group had centred on wanting to hide away from them!

The approach to DMT with children and adolescents is dependent upon the training and experience of the therapist as well as the context of the school itself. However, in my experience some general conclusions can be made about how to work with these groups. For example, the therapist needs to refrain from entering into an overtly authoritarian role with an aggressive and hostile group or the same pattern of conflict will emerge as previously in their lives. A low profile will yield a more positive transference. Joining the movement is important for these groups as well as for lethargic or highly anxious ones.

Some of the groups and individuals I have worked with did not have a positive movement attitude and this did limit the DMT process. The risk and inherent vulnerability for them of moving gave the message of 'I'm keeping closed off and uninvolved'. I am aware that I used anything to spark off a movement play attitude. For example, John was flicking his comb at the start of the session. Knowing how difficult it was for him to engage in movement I somehow managed to intervene and we played at throwing and catching the comb; having it fall off our sleeves and 'saving' it, in turn, spontaneously. This enabled a rapport to develop which was less threatening and focused on an object distanced enough for John to be able to engage in movement without realizing it. From that time on we had a trusting relationship in our sessions.

There are conclusions concerning the role of the therapist's own process as an indicator for the type of material which can be satisfactorily worked with by the client. My learning from the children and adolescents enabled a monitoring of their effects upon me. There is a potential for movement interaction between the client and therapist which is crucial to accept; the therapist needs to acknowledge what is hers in order to distinguish whose pathology is operating at any given moment (the client's or the therapist's).

The therapist's receptivity to the patient's unconscious communication [movement material] is manifest in his response to interactive pressures.

(Casement 1985: 95)

By self-reflection, personal therapy, and supervision the therapist can access a greater range of feeling. More than identifying empathically with what is familiar to their own experience, the therapist has to be able to develop a receptivity to feelings unlike their own. By recognizing the unfamiliar in the client more understanding of the client can result. For example, in the case of Steve his need for anger to be accepted by the therapist without retribution was important. Although his physical aggression towards others was always picked up as needing containing he was encouraged to express the anger through other means such as vigorous movement, drumming, and so on. In addition, by understanding the processes and issues underlying normal development, the therapist can be clearer on those dynamics which inhibit a satisfactory definition of self (in this material infant and adolescent development, and in particular that of the troubled and troublesome adolescent). For example, we can conclude that the conflict that is felt between love and hate directed against the same person needs to be satisfactorily regulated. 'The fear and guilt stemming from this conflict . . . and the inability to face the fear and guilt underlies much character disorder, including persistent delinquency' (Bowlby 1979: 5). The regulation of this ambivalence is crucial, directing and controlling contradictory impulses and developing a capacity to experience in a healthy manner the resulting anxiety and guilt. The fear of punishment expected from hostility (acts or intentions) leads to more aggression; guilt can demand demonstrations of love which, unmet, results in further hatred. If there is an unusually strong impulse to strive for a secure attachment or to hurt and destroy (even physically as in the case illustration) the very one who is loved, the regulation of the conflict will be more problematic.

It is helpful to have some awareness of both DMT research findings and psychotherapy research with the population in focus, particularly those links with psychotherapeutic and body-orientated theory. But it is the client who leads the therapist (who gently guides them with these kinds of signposts) from what they both know to what they still have to learn and understand. The client knows where they need to travel with the therapist's guidance; and by journeying together the therapist rediscovers theory from practice.

The notion of 'holding' (Winnicott 1971) or containment is crucial with these populations. As with physical holding there are many ways to do this to enable the client to discover their capacity to work through and manage conflicts without the need for 'fight or flight'. The establishment and maintenance of clear therapeutic boundaries such as ground rules and other therapeutic strategies discussed can provide for a level of containment which allows the therapist to survive the attacks and understand what is being encountered.

So what of the future for DMT with children and adolescents? Some of those with special educational needs will be placed in mainstream schools, those with the most disabling difficulties will be educated in special schools. Both types of school will be engaged in the national curriculum and be responsible for their own budgets. The implications for the rationale of DMT in special education of the arrival of these government innovations need to be carefully considered. The place of dance in the national curriculum is not clear, although there seems to be a move to include it within physical education again as it was over a decade ago. Dance is taught in special schools although it does not have a high status in the way arts and crafts or music do. Therefore, as with dance in mainstream education, the place of DMT will most likely be reflected by the place dance and movement education has on the curriculum; alternatively, it can find a home in the counselling service.

It is evident that those practitioners who have practised or are currently practising DMT in education have managed to do so as a result of goodwill as their schools recognize the value of the work. In my experience such posts, whether full or part time, fail to be replaced when practitioners leave. Until a proper career structure, conditions of service, salary, and union representation are provided for DMT in the education service this will continue[3]. DMT needs recognition as a profession in this service as a matter of urgency. In the meantime schools could employ a teacher trained in DMT which would make a positive contribution to dispelling the fears, myths, and misconceptions about dance movement therapy often occurring in the education system. If we believe in the need to have abilities to communicate, to make and maintain satisfactory relationships in the world, then DMT is applicable to all children and adolescents, as well as to those disturbed and disturbing or disabled and handicapped.

SUMMARY

This chapter has introduced a practice of DMT with children and adolescents within special education, the focus being on young people labelled delinquent. I have described issues as I have found them, offered through my own understanding. They are given for learning from not as a model.

ACKNOWLEDGEMENTS

I should like to send my appreciation to all the children and adolescents with whom I have worked and to colleagues.

NOTES

1 The 'conductor' is a technical term adopted for the facilitator in the group-analytic approach to group psychotherapy.
2 There is a move towards establishing the arts therapies as a separate profession within the education service. Further information may be obtained from the Arts Therapies in Education Committee, Chairperson, 115, Habberley Rd, Kidderminster, Worcs, DY1 15PW. A leaflet is being produced to enable employers to understand the role of the arts therapist in education and the different conditions of service required.
3 A pamphlet for heads and curriculum planners on dance in the national curriculum was produced in January 1990 and can be obtained from the Council for Dance Education and Training, 5, Tavistock Place, London WC1. The following areas are some which might be relevant to DMT in an educational context: personal and social education; artistic and aesthetic education; physical education, health, and fitness; and cross-curricular learning.

REFERENCES

Adelman, H. S. and Taylor, L. (1986) 'Children's reluctance regarding treatment: incompetence, resistance or an appropriate response', *School Psychology Review* 15(1): 91–9.
Adler, R. F. and Fisher, P. (1984) 'My self . . . through music, movement and

art', *Arts in Psychotherapy* 2(3): 203–8.

Ainsworth, M. D. S. (1962) 'The effects of maternal deprivation: a review of findings and controversy in the context of research strategy', in *Deprivation of Maternal Care: A Reassessment of its Effects*, Geneva: World Health Organization Public Health Papers, 14: 153.

Alvin, J. (1966) 'History of music therapy', in J. Alvin (1975) *Music Therapy*, London: Hutchinson.

Apter, A., Sharir, I., Tyano, S., and Wijsenbeck, H. (1978) 'Movement therapy with psychotic adolescents', *British Journal of Medical Psychology* 51(2): 155–9.

Balaz, S. E. (1977) *Dance Therapy in the Classroom*, New Jersey: Waldwick Hoctor Products for Education.

Barcai, A., Umbarger, C., Pierce, T. W., and Chamberlais, P. (1973) 'A comparison of three group approaches to underachieving children', *American Journal of Orthopsychiatry* 43(9): 133–41.

Berrol, C. F. (1989) 'A view from Israel: DMT and creative arts therapies in special education', *Arts in Psychotherapy* 16(2): 81–90.

Billington, H. (1981) 'Movement with disturbed children', *New Growth* 1(1): 43–7.

Bion, W. R. (1962) *Learning from Experience*, London: Heinemann.

Bowlby, J. (1951) *Maternal Care and Mental Health*, Monograph Series No: 2, second edition, Geneva: World Health Organization.

——(1979) *The Making and Breaking of Affectional Bonds*, London: Tavistock.

Bridgeways School (1985) 'Filling in the cracks', *Community Care* 11 April.

Britton, R. S. (1978) 'The deprived child', *The Practitioner* 221, September: 373–8.

Bruce, T. (1975) 'Adolescent groups and adolescent processes', *British Journal of Medical Psychology* 48: 333–8.

Bunt, L. (1986) 'Research in Great Britain into the effects of music therapy with particular reference to the child with a handicap', in E. Ruud (ed.) *Music and Health*, London: J. Chester.

Case, C. (1981) 'Problems with bereavement with maladjusted children', *Conference Proceedings*, Hertfordshire College of Art and Design, St Albans.

——(1986) 'Hide and seek: a struggle for meaning', in 'Looking at childhood', *Inscape* Winter.

——(1987) 'Loss and transition in art therapy with children', in T. Dalley, C. Case, J. Schaverien, F. Weir, D. Halliday, P. Nowell–Hall, and D. Waller, *Images of Art Therapy*, London: Tavistock.

——(1990) 'Reflections and shadows', in C. Case and T. Dalley (eds) *Working with Children in Art Therapy*, London: Routledge.

Casement, P. (1985) *On Learning from the Patient*, London: Routledge.

Cole, I. L. (1982) 'Movement negotiations with an autistic child', *Arts in Psychotherapy* 9(1): 49–53.

Creadick, T. A. (1985) 'The role of the expressive arts in therapy', *Journal of Reading, Writing and Learning Disabilities* 1(3): 55–60.

Curtis, M. and Gilmore, C. (1982) 'Group counselling in secondary schools', *Educational Psychology Journal*, 47–56.

Dalley, T. (1990) 'Images and integration: art therapy in a multi-cultural school', in C. Case and T. Dalley (eds) *Working with Children in Art Therapy*, London: Routledge.

Delany, W. (1973) 'Working with children', *Conference Proceedings*, 8th American Dance Therapy Association, Monograph 3.

De Martino, R. A. (1986) 'A meta analysis of school-based studies in psychotherapy', *Journal of School Psychology* 24: 3.

Dunne, C., Bruggen, P., and O'Brian, C. (1982) 'Touch and action in group therapy of younger adolescents', *Journal of Adolescence* 5: 31–8.

Eisler, R. M. and Frederikson, L. W. (1980) 'Perfecting social skills: a guide to therapeutic education', *Therapeutic Education* 1(1): 13–21.

Evans, J. (1980) 'Ambivalence and how to turn it to your advantage: adolescents and paradoxical intervention', *Journal of Adolescence* 3: 273–84.

Fisher, P. (1980) 'How a creative movement programme affects body image and self-concept in learning disabled children', *Scottish Journal of Physical Education* 8: 1.

Fisher, S and Cleveland, S. E. (1968) *Body Image and Personality*, New York: Dover Press.

Foulkes, S. H. (1965) *Therapeutic Group Analysis*, London: Allen & Unwin.

Foulkes, S. A. and Anthony, E. J. (1984) *Group Psychotherapy: The Psychoanalytic Approach*, London: Maresfield.

Freud, A. (1958) 'Adolescence', *Psychoanalytic Study of the Child* 13: 255–78.

——(1965) *Normality and Pathology in Childhood: Assessment of Development*, New York: International Universities Press.

Furman, L. (1990) 'Video therapy: an alternative for the treatment of adolescents', *Arts in Psychotherapy* 17: 165–9.

Graafsme, T. and Anbeck, M. (1984) 'Resistance in adolescence', *Journal of Adolescence* 7: 1–16.

Goodhill, S. (1987) 'Dance movement therapy with abused children', *Arts in Psychotherapy* 14(1): 59–68.

Groves, L. (1979) 'To dance with a smile; successful experience through dance', in L. Groves (ed.) *Physical Education for Special Needs*, Cambridge: Cambridge University Press.

Holmes, E. (1977) 'The educational needs of children in care', *Concern* 26: 22–5.

——(1980) 'Educational intervention for pre-school children in day or residential care', *Therapeutic Education* 8(2): 3–10.

——(1983) 'Psychological assessment', in M. Boston and R. Szur (eds) *Psychotherapy with Severely Deprived Children*, London: Routledge & Kegan Paul.

Hulton, D. (ed.) (1985) *The Arts for Young People with Special Needs: An Internal Report on the Carnegie Project 'Art for the Handicapped'*, Devon: Dartington College of Arts.

Jennings, S. (1973) *Remedial Drama*, London: Pitman.

Jennings, S. and Gersie, A. (1987), 'Drama therapy with disturbed adolescents', in *Dramatherapy: Theory and Practice for Teachers and Clinicians*, London: Routledge.

Johnson, D. R. and Eicher, V. (1990) 'The use of dramatic activities to facilitate dance therapy with adolescents', *Arts in Psychotherapy* 17: 157–64.

Kalish, B. I. (1968) 'Body movement therapy for autistic children', *Proceedings Conference American Dance Therapy Association*.

Kearne, F. (1978) 'Instructional models and the development of the body concept and anxiety reduction in elementary school children', Educational Report, Ohio University.

Kolvin, I., Garside, R. F., Nicol, A. R., Macmillan, A., Wolstenholme, F., and Leitch, I. (1981) *Help Starts Here: The Maladjusted Child in Ordinary School*, London: Tavistock.

Lacan, J. (1977) *The Four Fundamental Concepts of Psychoanalysis*, London: Hogarth Press.

Lasseter, J., Privette, G., Brown, C., and Duer, J. (1989) 'Dance as a treatment approach with a multi-disabled child: implications for school counselling', *School Counsellor* 36(4): 310–15.

Laufer, M. and Laufer, M. E. (1984) *Adolescence and Developmental Breakdown: A*

Psychoanalytical View, London and New Haven: Yale University Press.

Leste, A. and Rust, J. (1984) 'Effects of dance on anxiety', *Journal of Perceptual and Motor Skills* 58: 767–72.

Leventhal, M. (1974) 'Movement therapy with minimal brain dysfunction children', in K. Mason (ed.) *Focus on Dance Therapy*, Washington DC: American Alliance for Health, PE and Recreation.

——(1980) *Movement and Growth: Dance Therapy for the Special Child*, Proceedings from Symposium, New York University.

Lovell, S. M. (1980) 'The bodily-felt sense and body image changes in adolescence', in compendium of presenters *Abstracts of American Dance Therapy Association, 15th Annual Conference*.

McNeely, A. D. (1987) *Touching: Body Therapy and Depth Psychology*, Toronto: Inner City Books.

Marshall, R. (1982) 'The treatment of resistance in the psychotherapy of children and adolescents', *Psychotherapy: Theory, Research and Practice* 9(2), Summer.

Meekums, B. (1990) 'Dance movement therapy and the development of mother–child interaction', M.Phil. thesis, University of Manchester.

Meier, W. (1979) 'Meeting special needs through movement and dance drama', *Therapeutic Education* 7(1): 27–33.

Montague, A. (1971) *Touching*, New York: Columbia University Press.

Nicol, A. and Parker, J. (1981) 'Play group therapy in a junior school – 1: method and general problems', *British Journal of Guidance and Counselling* 9(1): 86–93 (and 2).

Nordoff, P. and Robbins, C. (1965) *Music Therapy for the Handicapped Child*, New York: Steiner Publishers.

North, M. (1972) *Personality Assessment through Movement*, London: Macdonald & Evans.

——(1973) *Movement Education*, London: Temple Smith.

Payne, H. (1981) 'Movement therapy for the special child', *British Journal of Dramatherapy* 4: 3.

——(1984) 'Responding with dance', *Maladjustment and Therapeutic Education* 2(2): 42–57.

——(1985) 'Jumping for joy', *Changes Journal of Psychology and Psychotherapy* 3(4): 25–8.

——(1986) 'Dance movement therapy with male adolescents labelled delinquent – a pilot study', *Conference Proceedings, VIIIth Commonwealth and International Conference on Sport, P.E., Dance, Recreation and Health; Dance: The Study and the Place of Dance in Society*, London: E. and F. N. Spon.

——(1987) 'The perceptions of male adolescents labelled delinquent towards a programme of dance movement therapy', M.Phil. thesis, University of Manchester.

——(1988a) 'The practice of dance movement therapy with adolescents', *Conference Proceedings: Dance and the Child International*, London: Roehampton Institute.

——(1988b) 'The use of dance movement therapy with troubled youth', in C. Schaefer (ed.) *Innovative Interventions in Child and Adolescent Therapy*, New York/London: John Wiley Interscience.

——(1990) *Creative Movement and Dance in Groupwork*, Oxon: Winslow.

Pfeifer, G. and Spinner, D. (1985) 'Combined individual and group psychotherapy with children: an ego development perspective', *International Journal of Group Psychotherapy* 35(1): 11–35.

Pines, M. (1982) 'Reflections on mirroring', *Group Analysis* 15(2): 1–26.

Rabiochow, M. G. and Sklansky, M. D. (1980) *Effective Counselling of Adolescents*, Chicago: Follett.

Rakusin, A. (1990) 'A dance/movement therapy model incorporating movement education concepts for emotionally disturbed children', *The Arts in Psychotherapy* 17: 55–67.

Rogers, S. B. (1977) 'Contributions of dance therapy in the treatment of retarded adolescents and adults', *Arts Psychotherapy* 4(3–4): 195–7.

Rutter, M. L. and Giller, H. (1982) *Juvenile Delinquency: Trends and Perspectives*, London: Guilford Press.

Scott, R. (1988) 'An investigation into the outcomes of dance and movement in the curriculum of children with emotional and behavioural difficulties', *Conference Proceedings, Second Arts Therapies Research*, London: City University.

Shennum, W. A. (1987) 'Expressive activity therapy in residential treatment', *Child and Youth Care Quarterly* 16(2): 81–90.

Sherborne, V. (1975) 'Movement for retarded and disturbed children', in S. Jennings (ed.) *Creative Therapy*, London: Pitman.

——(1990) *Developmental Movement for Children*, Cambridge: Cambridge University Press.

Shuttleworth, R. (1981) 'Adolescent dramatherapy', in G. Shattner and R. Courtney (eds) *Drama in Therapy*, Vol. 2, New York: Drama Books.

Siegel, E. V. (1973) 'Movement therapy with autistic children', *The Psychoanalytic Review* 60: 1.

Slaveson, S. R. and Schiffer, M. (1975) *Group Psychotherapies for Children*, New York: International Universities Press.

Spielberger, C. (1983) *Manual for the State-Trait Anxiety Inventory (Form Y)*, Palo Alto, CA: Consulting Psychologists Press.

Stern, D. N. (1974) 'Mother and infant at play: the dydadic interaction involving facial, vocal and gaze behaviour', in M. Lewis and L. A. Rosenblum (eds) *The Effect of the Infant on its Caregiver*, New York: Wiley.

——(1985) *The Interpersonal World of the Infant*, New York: Basic Books.

Tipple, B. (1975) 'Dance therapy and education', *Journal of Leisurability* 2(4): 9–12.

Truax, C. B. and Carkuff, R. (1967) *Toward Effective Counselling and Psychotherapy*, Chicago: Aldine.

Watts, A. (1973) *Psychotherapy East and West*, Harmondsworth, Middx: Pelican.

Wheeler, B. (1987) 'The use of paraverbal therapy in treating an abused child', *Arts in Psychotherapy*, 14(1): 69–76.

Wiener, J. and Helbraun, E. (1985) 'Creative movement with the learning disabled child', *Journal of Reading, Writing and Learning Disabilities* 1(3): 34–44.

Wilson and Evans (1980) *The Education of Disturbed Pupils*, The Schools Council Working Paper 65.

Willis, C. (1987) 'Legal and ethical issues of touch in dance/movement therapy', *American Journal of Dance Therapy* 10: 41–53.

Winnicott, D. W. (1962) 'Ego integration in child development', in *The Maturational Processes and the Facilitating Environment*, London: Hogarth Press and the Institute of Psycho-Analysis, 1965.

——(1971) *Playing and Reality*, London: Tavistock.

Wislochi, A. (1981) 'Movement is their medium: DMT in special education', *Milieu Therapy* 1(1): 49–54.

Chapter 4

Older lives, older dances
Dance movement therapy with older people

Susan Stockley

INTRODUCTION

The culture of ageing

During the last thirty years or more an increasing number of people are surviving beyond retirement age. In Britain, 16 per cent of the population are now elderly (over 65 years old), and by the year 2,000 this figure will have grown to 20 per cent (Comfort 1977). By this time there will also be a 40 per cent increase in the number of people aged over 85 years. Thus with more over 60s in the community more services will be required to meet their needs, whether they are living alone, with family, or in sheltered or institutionalized accommodation.

It is worth noting, particularly for the purposes of applying dance movement therapy, that old age is a growth stage in its own right. The perceived needs of older people are very much affected by ageism in our society. Ageism refers to:

> the pejorative image of someone who is 'old' simply because of his/her age . . . it is wholesale discrimination against all members of this category. Cutbacks in social security, failure to provide meaningful outlets or activities, or the belief that those in their 60s and beyond do not benefit from psychotherapy are all examples of subtle, or in some cases not so subtle appraisals of the old. Part of the myth, a fundamental if implicit element of ageism, is the view that the elderly are somehow different from our present and future selves, and therefore not subject to the same desires, concerns or fears.
>
> (Hendricks and Hendricks 1977: 177)

At 65 or 60 men and women are subjected to compulsory unemployment by the state, leading to subsequent loss of income, activity, and status. Their condition is further worsened by the probable loss of fitness and health, and by bereavement and isolation.

A dance movement therapist who chooses to work with older people will probably do so in the context of social, educational, and health services offered to elderly people by public and charitable organizations. These services will be operating within a culture which has ageist attitudes, and that demeans and denigrates the old whilst idolizing beauty, youthfulness, and the future. An important aspect of the work done by a dance movement therapist will lie in combating ageism, particularly at the level at which older people have themselves internalized it. Many older people engage in self-debasement, hating themselves and their lives and the company of their peers, feeling they are worthless and there is nothing left to live for. As Tony Ward has noted with regard to the images of ageing:

> Negative and discriminatory stereotyping is widely practised on TV and in the media, and can have considerable ill-effects not just on attitudes towards the elderly, but also on the self-perception of the elderly themselves.
>
> (Ward 1989: 8)

Ageism is very much influenced by the way in which issues of dependency in the elderly are negatively regarded in our culture, particularly during the Thatcherite era of anti-dependency values. This is most clearly seen in the attitudes of those who are not yet old themselves, in expressions such as 'wrinklies' or 'old dodderers'. Because an older person may not physically be able to do all the things they could twenty years earlier, such as drive a car or paint the ceiling, that person is seen as incompetent and dependent by relatives, social services, and the GP, for example, simply because they require some help with travelling or decorating. Phyllida Salmon, who has written on this subject, believes that 'by defining the old as dependent, we apparently make them comparable with children . . . and yet our views of their two kinds of dependency are not the same' (Salmon 1985: 36).

Physical support is gladly given to the dependent young, whereas it tends to be given grudgingly to the dependent old. Salmon thinks that this has something to do with 'the fact that the old have a long past, while the young have a long future'. Future potential in the young is more highly valued than a lifetime of past experiences in the old, which are seen as obsolete. The needs of the very dependent elderly are contained in institutions where they can be kept alive until it is time to die. Under these conditions dependency needs are multiplied by the loss of personal identity and autonomy, and by the feeling that life is nothing but a grey, anonymous existence. When life has reached this stage elders really do need positive input from society as a whole to counteract the negativity of existing in a shrunken life space, which may feel more like a prison or place of abandonment than a warm and safe home.

Another perspective is to realize that ignoring the past impoverishes the present. Perhaps if more of the past was integrated into the present in people's lives, the future would n̂ot have to be either dreaded or idealized. One way of valuing older people's unique contribution to our society is to regard them, as Salmon says, 'as a witness, a witness of what has been', both of their individual pasts and of the eras through which they have lived. Dance movement therapy can be an important part of this process of endorsing past life experiences, and of communicating and integrating them.

Historical overview

With an increasingly ageing population which is no longer in employment, and with the breakdown of the extended family and the emergence of the Welfare State at the end of the Second World War, various structures have been designed by social services and the National Health Service to try to contain the needs of older people. Day centre provision and occupational therapy programmes are examples of care which was originally designed to rehabilitate the sick or chronically disabled elderly, and so prevent long-term hospitalization or institutionalized care.

During the 1960s and 1970s several different organizations pioneered the beginnings of the use of arts activities and arts therapies with various disadvantaged populations. In 1976, Gina Levete, a dancer, founded SHAPE which took creative arts into homes for the elderly, hospitals, and day centres. SESAME was working even earlier than this, using drama and movement therapeutically in hospitals and day centres. Prior to this, advocates of Rudolf von Laban's theories of movement and educational and creative dance, such as Audrey Wethered (1976) and Chloe Gardner (with Wethered, 1987), had applied these ideas therapeutically in hospitals, mainly with psychiatric and psycho-geriatric patients. Other organizations, such as EXTEND, also took recreative movement into homes and hospitals for the elderly. The use of art, music, and drama as therapies was more established than the use of dance and movement, but the acceptance of the former in psychiatric institutions and day centres for people with learning difficulties had paved the way for dance movement therapy to get on its feet. With the promotion of equal opportunities policies in education and social services, older people began to gain a higher profile, at least in terms of their needs, and the provision of classes and programmes specifically for elders became established.

Thus the social and cultural settings in which DMT with older people takes place are to be found in day and community centres, in hospitals and homes for the elderly. The working contract between the dance movement therapist and the client group may come from social services adult education special needs departments, or occasionally occupational therapy departments in NHS hospitals. Employers' expectations may range from physical and emotional rehabilitation to enhancement of the quality of life for the participants. As for the clients themselves, they may hope for greater mobility and improved general health, higher self-esteem, and to reap the benefits of mutual support and interaction.

In general, working with elders has had less status both in training and in practice, the greater focus having been on psychiatric patients, physical and mental handicap, and work with 'special' children. The choices of DMT students in special studies bear this out. It seems that both in training and in practice ageism is at work again.

Models and approaches

In Britain very little has been written about either recreational movement or dance movement therapy with elders. What is available takes the form of short articles or chapters in an arts therapies publication or a few articles circulated only to practitioners, for example, Pasch (1982). No in-depth research studies have been published. The main documented theoretical background for dance movement therapy with elders comes from American publications. Dance movement therapy in the United States is twenty to thirty years in advance of the current situation in Britain.

The British Association for Dance Movement Therapy defines dance movement therapy as 'the use of expressive movement and dance as a medium through which the individual can engage creatively in a process of personal integration and growth' (ADMT 1989),[1] which means that the aims and methods of dance movement therapy are quite distinct from the use of creative movement and fitness programmes. Whereas fitness or dance sessions might aim to improve mobility, circulation, and breathing, emotional well-being is seen more as a by-product than a goal. Dance movement therapy programmes seek to integrate physiological, psychological, and sociological elements, and give meaning to movement through the development of images within the movement interaction. Movement activities are not the goal of the experience, but the tool for creating a therapeutic environment.

Another important difference lies in the quality of the relationship between the teacher (or therapist) and the students (or clients). In the teaching of many forms of dance and keep fit the teachers often adopt a 'Simon Says' style which reinforces their power as experts and essentially invalidates the students themselves as individuals with specific contributions to make, effectively keeping them at a distance. A dance movement therapist will take a more creative and empathic stance, which empowers and validates the participants' individual experiences. The therapist is 'with' the clients, on all the levels that human movement involves: the physical or mechanical, the communicative or expressive, and the symbolic or unconscious aspects, whether physically moving with them or in the role of observer.

DMT with elders was started in America as early as 1942, when Marian Chace (Chaiklin 1975) began working with psychiatric and elderly patients at St Elizabeth's Hospital in Washington, DC. Her main technique consisted of empathic improvised movement. Sandel and Read refer to this as:

> a technique in which the therapist guides and develops group interaction as it unfolds during the session. . . . The therapist creates an atmosphere that encourages self-expression through movement. This technique challenges the therapist's skill in dealing with spontaneous movement expressions and group processes.
>
> (Sandel and Read 1987: 28)

Susan Sandel also developed a group-orientated, interactional approach with elders, focusing on the psycho-social benefits to the participants at a specialized care centre. Sandel developed her approach in the 1950s and 1960s, and found that the following specific techniques provided a sound and beneficial structure for DMT programmes with elders: the use of a circular formation, mutual touch, music, vocalization, props, empathic movement, imagery, and reminiscing. Sandel maintained that the circle is the primary spatial form for interaction and contact, and is a good way to begin and end sessions. She found that mutual touch encourages people t᷄ reach out to one another, provides sensory stimulation, and facilitates emotional contact. Music can help to engender a feeling of group unity, particularly through rhythm, the creation of atmosphere, or the invocation of a memory. Vocalization can enlarge movement and the expression of feelings. Props can help to develop a movement quality such as stretching or pushing, and stimulate activity and interaction. Empathic movement will involve the therapist supporting, intervening in, and challenging what the clients express. The use of imagery shifts the experience from that of a simple action to that of a symbolic shared act, as the image develops out of the movement. In reminiscence, the same approach applies: the progression is from a sensory experience (movement) to a symbolic one (association from the past). Reminiscing can be a behavioural adaptation to growing older, and dance movement therapy can encourage and enhance this process.

A third American dance movement therapist who developed a

specialized approach to work with older people is Eva Desca Garnet. Garnet found that 'because the physical aspects of ageing are so pronounced, I use a somatic rather than a psychological emphasis in geriatric movement therapy' (Garnet 1982: 15) Garnet seems to believe that the psychological issues faced by the elderly, which might include fear of dependence, bereavement and loss, death or abandonment, are best addressed through dealing with the somatic results of ageing, such as disease, injury, and sensory loss. Garnet gives the following outline of how her approach, which is the product of twelve years' work and research, helps elders to meet their needs.

1 By supplementing movement and sensory deficit, a physiological need is fulfilled.
2 By the physical safety of the movement, and the psychological safety of the presentation, an ego need for security is filled.
3 By promoting a feeling of group consciousness that grows out of a helping relationship, a feeling of belonging is achieved.
4 By promoting a congenial supportive environment in which a group laughs easily at the same things, a participant changes his frame of reference from fatigue and depression to relaxation and exhilaration.
5 By acceptance and accommodation of each person's limitations, an atmosphere is created which facilitates the recognition of each person's unique achievements.

(Garnet 1974)

TECHNIQUES

In order to develop an understanding of which dance movement therapy techniques are the most appropriate to use in work with elders, we need to look more closely at the important therapeutic issues with this population.

Therapeutic issues

An older body and psyche have a longer history than a younger person; there is more on the map, with probably both more strengths and more weaknesses. The older normal neurotic/schizoid person, who has not had any major mental illnesses requiring long-term drug treatment or hospitalization, will have developed many coping and compensatory patterns evident in both physical and emotional structure and functioning. Those patterns will no doubt have served a particular senior citizen very well through a lifetime of working, child rearing, and trying to gain some self-fulfilment. Older people will have survived one or two world wars and will know about struggle, hope, disappointment, and loss.

The physical changes of ageing have been well documented by geriatricians. Tissue regeneration slows down and there is a gradual deterioration in the functioning of all the organs and systems of the body. Most medical specialists regard these changes, which are termed 'senescence', as normal and not pathological. The observable and measurable bodily changes consist of the following:

1 bones become thinner and eventually osteoporotic. This occurs more quickly in women because of the loss of the calcium-maintaining oestrogens after the menopause. Cartilege and disc material also shrinks and is less able to buffer the bones;
2 the skin becomes thinner and less elastic, with fewer fat and nerve cells, less protection and more bruising;
3 the respiratory system becomes less efficient, particularly as the arteries shrink and harden;
4 cardiac and voluntary muscle becomes smaller, less effective, slower, weaker, and less able to regenerate;
5 brain weight decreases and brain cells die and are not replaced;
6 the kidneys' filtering system becomes less effective;
7 the sensations of touch, taste, and smell decrease with age.

Most of the descriptive words used by geriatricians and biologists to describe ageing are to do with deterioration: thinning, wrinkling, shrinking, impairment, atrophy, degeneration. This view tends to write off all physical illnesses as problems that older people inevitably experience due to the process of ageing, what might be called the 'it's your age dear' or 'what do you expect at your age?' syndrome. However, other studies challenge the view of inevitable deterioration and state that:

> While all these changes of ageing are well known, we do not really know how much is due to the ageing process itself and how much results from our sedentary lifestyle . . . physical inactivity can make a body age prematurely.
>
> (Leventhal 1988: 3)

Deterioration in physical functioning is partly the result of the lack of physical activity which gives rise to what are termed hypo-kinetic disorders.

Application

With the physiological issues of ageing looming so large and evoking feelings of fear, frustration, and resignation in many people, it does make sense for dance movement therapy programmes with older people to address the somatic issues of mobility, strength, flexibility, co-ordination, and respiratory and cardio-vascular fitness. We all live both in and through our bodies, and our sense of psychological well-being and wholeness is profoundly affected by our body image and physical capacities. Unnecessary loss through outward neglect or internalized negativity does not make for self-respect or a positive sense of health. Marcia Leventhal, an American dance therapist, believes that for elders 'a dance movement therapy programme must pay attention to the physiological parameters of aging and offer movement experiences which will help to alleviate some of the functional losses' (Leventhal 1988: 8). On this aspect she agrees with Eva Desca Garnet that the physical problems are real and important. Garnet describes what she regards as the paradox of old age as 'inactivity versus health'. 'In the life cycle there is an increasingly emotional distance between the early ecstacy of movement, and the later period when it can scarcely be endured. Yet the biological need for activity is ever present' (Garnet 1974: 59). Even where disease and injury are present, prolonged resting and inactivity only heighten discomfort.

One of the results of inactivity and a lack of movement and body awareness can be what Garnet describes as a 'postural set', evident in many older people, characterized by the contracture of the unused muscles and ligaments that connect the bony framework. This can lead to stooping, a shuffling gait, a fear of falling, and a body that moves with great distress. The postural set will sometimes be a further exaggeration of a person's earlier physical and psychological character structure, which might, in terms of the categories developed by a somatic psychologist, Stanley Kelleman (1985), be either rigid, dense, swollen, or collapsed. The act of having to face one's lifelong restrictions and compensations as an older person gives rise to fresh opportunities for evaluation, integration, and change.

Many of the psychological theories around ageing are themselves ageist, or, as Gordon Lowe says, 'adultomorphic prejudices are almost universally taken for granted, tacitly assumed by most investigators of old age, and helplessly shared by many old people themselves' (Lowe 1976: 244).

This means that older people are not seen as capable of change, but as degenerated, helpless, and as second- or third-class citizens. Lowe reminds us that 'Psychology tends to be so over-impressed with the negative implications of biology, that the positive features of old age have tended to be ignored or denied' (Lowe 1976: 245). Many of the myths are social or sexual. For example, there is the view that retirement at 65 years of age equals social death or that after the menopause sexuality dies off along with fertility in women, or that sexual activity in the older man means being a dirty old man. Another negatively stereotypical view put forward by Cumming and Henry (1961) was that ageing is a process of disengagement of older people from their society, and that this process is inevitable and even desirable. During this disengagement the elderly would seem to fall into a sort of limbo or second childhood with the expectation that their grown-up children, or institutional carers, will do all the looking after necessary, and make all the decisions for them.

In Erik Erikson's (1977) developmental model of the psychology of growing through life, from birth to death, the issue to be faced in the last stage is 'Integrity versus despair'. This implies that a good experience of the last years is very dependent on how problems have been dealt with at previous stages, such as the penultimate stage called 'Generativity versus stagnation'. In the face of failure and stuckness it may be difficult to find integrity, and easy to feel that despair and hopelessness are all that remain. Marcia Leventhal believes:

> The psychology of the senior adult is reminiscent of the emerging infant's stages of separation and individuation, only in reverse. As the life-space experiential world shrinks due to loss – loss of friends and family, and physical faculties and capabilities, so the senior seems to be exhibiting a strong need for a more dependent symbiotic union with his environment.
>
> (Leventhal 1988: 3)

Elderly people may cling to their grown-up children, or become almost autistic and unable to respond to help or stimulation, so that helping them to find a balance between dependence and autonomy seems to be an important issue. Help that was not required before may now be needed, for example after a stroke, but the person still needs to feel independent and adult. Perhaps the biggest and most profound issue that most older adults have to deal with is that of loss, not only of physical health and mental faculties, and of loved ones and family, but of a working life that provided a structure for living. Older people may feel that their lives have shrunk or fallen apart and that they are just waiting for death. Making activities such as dance movement therapy available for the older population can help to provide a structure and possibly a meaning to living out one's final years of life.

Probably the most difficult loss to deal with is severe sensory impairment such as deafness, blindness or partial sight, loss of speech, and loss of skin sensation. These kinds of sensory impairment can be the direct result of illnesses such as cataracts, tinnitis, strokes, multiple sclerosis, and Parkinson's disease. The use of sensory stimulation as an intervention in dance movement therapy can be of particular use here. Sensory stimulation provokes a response kinaesthetically which helps balance spatial orientation, so that a person feels more grounded in the here and now, and more self-aware. Emotionally, sensory stimulation provides contact, warmth, and closeness, and decreases a person's sense of isolation and despair. The need to experience warm, loving contact continues throughout life; it is not a prerogative of babies and young lovers. The contact needs to be caring, with respect for the older person's wishes, and not invasive.

Dance movement therapy is an appropriate choice and has a special place in helping populations which have sensory loss and difficulty with verbal or intellectual insight – and many of the older frail elderly come into this category – for example, by maintaining the integrity of the body image, the ego, and self-image. It can also provide a much needed sense of belonging and purpose, and an opportunity for validating past life experience, bringing them into the present as real contributions.

Practical aspects

Most DMT sessions with older people take place in a specific care-type setting, such as a community or day centre, hospital or residential home. There have been attempts to train care staff, at least in exercise and creative movement, but having tutors and therapists come in from outside seems to be preferable. According to some research done in the London Borough of Hackney, 'it was overwhelmingly preferred to have outside tutors . . . take movement sessions rather than in house staff . . . a different person coming in to take sessions created a certain interest in the activity' (Keatinge 1989: 73). It was also recognized that if the sessions were to be taken seriously by all concerned they needed to be done by an expert, so that they are not just seen as a frivolous extra or a way of passing the time.

Another aspect of having DMT taken seriously is to have all supervision and equipment, such as a tape cassette or props, paid for by the employer. It is very important to have time built into the work for talking to care staff and project managers about the clients and their progress, and problems such as the need for more privacy for the group or more care staff input. This is not the same as supervision, which is best done with a dance movement or arts trained therapist, or with a psychotherapist. The need for a relationship with carers and managers is a form of ongoing public relations and gives the work a higher profile and greater credibility.

When the clients actively choose to come to DMT sessions on a regular basis it makes progression possible. Sometimes clients are herded in by care staff twenty to thirty at a time on the premise that 'what's good for one is good for all', or just so that the care staff can get a break themselves. A dance movement therapist needs to be very clear about boundaries and commitment; for example, making the space into a safe and containing place, or being clear about the minimum and maximum number of group members and their regular attendance, and being aware that movement is a physical medium having definite ground rules around not hurting oneself, others, or property. Back-up from a professional organization or trade union may be necessary to ensure adequate working conditions, along with professional insurance if working privately.

An example of a structure for sessions

Sessions need to take place in a warm and friendly environment, a safe space where there will not be unnecessary interruptions or intrusions. Participants are encouraged to wear comfortable, loose clothing in which they will not feel inhibited or constrained. (This may be a problem for older women always used to wearing skirts.) Through movement and dance these older adults will be encouraged to find a greater range of movement and expression, and to explore their physical, mental, emotional, and social capabilities. A balance of moving, interacting, communicating, talking, and reflecting needs to be incorporated into the session. Senior citizens' past life experiences need to be validated and accepted. This helps to create an empathic and non-judgemental environment in which the need for change and its active process can be addressed in a way which is safe. The physiological health of elders needs to be addressed too, as the experience of chronic physical ill health can trigger off depression and withdrawal even in a previously coping and well-adjusted person. Improving and maintaining physical performance, particularly in terms of alignment and posture, and the functioning of the circulatory and respiratory systems, will encourage mental and emotional health, and mean that the physical body can help to support and integrate emotional changes.

Ideally, the structure for dance movement therapy sessions for people over sixty will contain the following parts.

1 Warm-up

This is usually done whilst seated in chairs in a circle. Introduction may be done verbally and through movement (such as passing a movement or an object around the circle). The aim of this exercise is to help people to arrive fully; to be in the session physically, mentally, and emotionally. Focusing on breathing and doing gentle movements with all the body parts, to articulate and sense kinaesthetically all the parts of the self, assists basic body awareness and people's arrival process. Self-massage can also be used as part of this process.

2 Thematic preparation

In this section larger, whole body movements are encouraged, so that people expand and stretch themselves and use the space more fully. All participants are encouraged to contribute a movement, that is, to initiate a movement which can be followed and shared by everyone in the group. A group rhythm will probably develop from this sharing process, so that people have a sense of belonging and of being an individual. Some participants may need the help of others or some support from chairs to maintain mobility or uprightness. Various types of movements and qualities may emerge from this section such as swaying, pushing, stamping, twisting, turning, stepping, swinging, etc. The choice of these actions, and the way in which they are executed, will reflect individual movement preferences and styles, as well as the moods and feelings of the moment. The aim is for material and energy to be stirred up and brought out in this section. Music may be used, for example, strong rhythmic music if the group looks ready to start off this way or a gentler waltz to coax people to move in a way that is relaxed and fluid. During this time the therapist will be observing as fully as possible all that is happening, and probably taking part as well, in order to get a clear idea of what the movement material is and how it can be developed and worked with later in the session.

3 Resting and sharing

This is an opportunity for the participants to rest physically and notice any changes in themselves, such as increased heart rate, expanded respiration, and how the parts of their bodies have responded to moving. Some people may really have liked the feeling of moving and dancing with others, whereas other people may have found the contact a bit overwhelming and want to withdraw. Heightened body- and self-awareness can be very revealing, particularly when overcoming a disability or chronic problem. People may also reminisce about movement memories and feelings from the past or express something that is going on in their lives right now. Sometimes this part of the session is done in pairs (especially if it is a large group), or through listening to each other in a small group. Sometimes a little self-massage is done, to help relax the body and encourage interchange.

4 Developing the theme

This is the time when the group will work more specifically with movements which emerged during the second section. People will be encouraged to let go more fully into the dynamics of a movement, for example, to intensify the movement and feeling of swaying or rocking in order to find out what memories and emotions these movements evoke. Sometimes this process can be enhanced by working in pairs and mirroring or providing mutual support, or by exchanging partial body weight support. A prop such as a ball or rope can help to enlarge or focus a movement. It can be useful, when the individuals in the group are familiar with each other and feel safe, to have one or two people moving in the centre of the space, with the others providing support through linking together or clapping or somehow echoing the central person's rhythm. The supporting movers can offer feedback that can be useful, insightful, and sometimes confrontative. For example, it may be observed that a woman in the centre of the circle does not contact the ground as strongly with her left foot as she does with her right. Although we can see that she is right-handed and right-sided, there is a sense of the left side being very protected, and so she is given this feedback. In response she may say that she broke her left ankle thirty years ago, but was totally unaware that her two feet now moved differently. The therapist and group may suggest that she try sensing the ground more with her left foot, trusting it and taking more risks. The restriction may have affected other aspects of her posture and movement as well, and psychologically reveal a tendency for caution and protection. In addition, other memories of what happened thirty years ago for her may emerge. Finally, in this section, as in the second, there may also be opportunities for people simply to enjoy dancing together for the pleasure it brings.

5 Relaxation and closure

This is an opportunity for people to release physical and emotional tensions and learn how to relax the body and mind totally, so that healing and integration can take place. There may be work with breathing, progressive relaxation of all body parts, and the use of imagery and visualization. People may also share their experiences verbally during this time of slowing down and coming back into reality.

This structure is really a model one which would have to be adapted to the needs of different groups. It may take several months or even years for a group to be able to access all five parts. A group of elders with very severe disabilities and impairment may need a great deal of help from music and props and from care staff able to offer one-to-one support. Such clients may be able to work only through sections one, two, and five.

CASE ILLUSTRATION

It is important for therapists to know why they have chosen to work with a particular client group, so that underlying transference and counter-transference issues can become clear, and the mutuality of the working relationship be safely explored. In my own case, from doing a mixture of special needs adult education work with students with learning difficulties, sessions at psychiatric day centres, and work with various older groups from different cultural and racial backgrounds, I gradually gravitated towards doing more work with older people. In particular, I found myself working mainly with older women and those of a specific ethnic origin or class identity, such as working-class women and Afro-Caribbean first-generation immigrants. I feel this choice was connected with my own process of rapidly growing up into an older and more grounded woman myself, and also wanting to have a healing relationship with the older (my parents') generation. I have also felt drawn to working with stroke patients and older people who have experienced bereavement, mutually learning about how much of life is about coming to terms with loss creatively. My approach includes working with body image using movement, creative dance, and the Feldenkrais method[2] within a psychotherapeutic framework.

An Afro-Caribbean group

The group I want to talk about has been in existence for nearly six years (at least as an open rather than a closed group). They are Afro-Caribbean senior citizens, mainly women, although the ratio of men has increased. I have a contract to do movement and dance for between thirty-two and forty weeks of the year on a regular weekday morning. My contract came through the local adult education institute's special needs department, following a request from the senior citizens' project concerned. The course first ran for a trial ten weeks and quickly became well subscribed. My first impression of this group, initially of about ten women, was that they were natural and expressive movers and, at an age between 60 and 75, very mobile. I was rather apprehensive about being a white person coming in to lead a group of black women in movement. After all, they moved extremely well and could probably teach me a few things! In those first few sessions it quickly became evident that we both shared a great joy in dancing together.

At the same time I realized there seemed to be an attraction of opposites or differences. They were Afro-Caribbean immigrants, over 60 and had long histories of working and parenting. In Laban terms their main movement 'effort' preferences were for weight and time (North 1972: 231). I was white and English, about half their age, with less experience of work and none at all in parenting or immigration, and my effort preferences, at that time, were for space and flow. In theoretical terms, if a mutual exchange of energy and movement patterns could take place, then we would all learn to access a wider range of effort movement qualities. According to Rudolf von Laban, the four motion factors discernible in all human movement are space, weight, flow, and time. We all have inner attitudes to these motion factors and some attitudes are more conscious than others. Space refers to the way the body uses space, and to spatial orientation; it is very much a thinking quality. Weight has to do with the use of body weight, and of sensation and grounding. Flow reflects the continuity of a movement and is also to do with the flow of energy through the body. Time has to do with decision-making and intuition. Laban's four elements of motion can be compared with Jung's typology of personality with its four functions of thinking, sensation, feeling, and intuition, where one of the aims of psychotherapeutic work is consciously to have access to all four functions.

Another characteristic of this Afro-Caribbean group of women, in addition to their solidity and strong rhythmic sense, is their religious faith, which was a strong influence on them during their upbringing in the West Indies. In the last couple of centuries this faith gave black people the strength to survive and fight slavery and domination. Here, in this country now, it seems to serve the purpose of strengthening their individual and collective fight against racism and oppression. As one member of the group wrote in a published collection of older women's memories at work, 'we were taught at school to call Britain the Mother Country', but when responding to advertisements offering accommodation, she recalled, 'As soon as the door was open and the colour was obvious, the door would be slammed shut in our faces' (Stanley 1989: 70).

A few of the women have recently been converted to the Pentecostal faith, probably in order to renew their spiritual energies and find strength and identity in the midst of a disorientating multi-cultural life with racism and oppression. I believed that the dance and movement group could be a place where these women would be able to validate their essential nature and differences from the white host culture, and also find out how to offset some of the problems they face in their daily lives, such as isolation, poverty, and discrimination, as well as disease and chronic illness.

One of the first characteristics that I noticed in relation to myself as leader of this group was their deference to me as the expert. This was not a role I wanted to be in or to encourage, partly because I felt it could reinforce and reflect the existing power imbalance between black and white so present in our society. No one in the group had been a teacher or leader themselves. People had worked in various low-paid jobs in the National Health Service, in factories, and in public transport, work where they were put in their place and told what to do. The project co-ordinator was also keen for me to encourage these pensioners to take responsibility for themselves and to make informed choices. Doris, the co-ordinator, saw retirement as a time for life's opportunities to open out, rather than shrink and diminish. So early on I encouraged group members to find their own movements, their natural bodily expression, and to initiate and lead each other with less reliance on me. Once given the opportunity, and the initial guidance, people soon learned to do this, and many very expressive and dynamic movements emerged which at first I had some difficulty in following, because they felt strange to me. In my spare time I decided to learn African dance in order to find in my own body the roots of these women's movements. From years of stretching, reaching, and trying to overcome gravity through the techniques of dance I had learned, such as ballet, contemporary dance, and even yoga, I found myself yielding more to gravity, in stronger contact with the ground and with my sexuality, and more in tune with these women. At the same time they frequently asked me to teach them 'your movements'. They were eager to learn yoga type stretches and movements which travelled through space and off the ground, such as long runs and jumps and flowing waltzes, which were less familiar to them. A process of mutual exchange had started.

Two years on from the start of the group, and of the pensioners' project itself, the project co-ordinator became involved in a political crisis to do with funding and fighting racism and embezzlement of funds in the local council. Pensioners who came to the project as a whole became divided between supporting the project co-ordinator or the local councillors involved. The supporters of the project co-ordinator were all members of the group, and together we decided to invite Doris to come to the group whenever possible for encouragement and help in dealing with the crisis creatively. The ten women actively campaigned for their worker and for the project to receive continued funding. I, as leader of the group, felt moved by their commitment, and assisted their cause by, amongst other things, writing letters and signing their petition. At this time a special ritual emerged in the group; it was someone's idea to sing a hymn together as a way of finding power and strength in a small group. We sang and moved to the chorus of the hymn 'Bind us together Lord':

> Bind us together Lord,
> Bind us together with cords that cannot be broken.
> Bind us together Lord,
> Bind us together Lord,
> Bind us together with Love.

This ritual of prayer in song and movement, with which the group likes to start each session, seems to express solidarity, strength of feeling and of faith, both in a God and in each other. The combination of spiritual expression through song and movement that I have shared with these people reminded me of my past involvement with a liturgical dance group. This was an appropriate form of expression for me at a certain time of my life, as in the Afro-Caribbean group, spiritual and expressive content is an appropriate form for its members' situation now.

I would like to talk about two members of the group, women who are the only remaining original members from six years ago.

Celia

Celia is in her mid-70s and an extremely solid and grounded older woman. Her predominant movement style shows a slow, undulating, rhythmic quality with a lot of enjoyment of her body and her sexuality. Underneath this there is sometimes a shadow movement which suggests a kind of self-contained pushing away, which says something like 'I'm really OK, you know'. In her commitment to the project and the group Celia has been extremely solid and consistent; I cannot remember her ever missing a session. When I was pregnant and still taking the group, the subject of having children and mothering came up. I had made stereotypical assumptions (drawn from the women's generally rounded size and movements), that it was normal for all of these Afro-Caribbean older women to be natural Earth Mothers. As a pregnant woman I enjoyed having my tummy patted each week by many of them to check my baby's growth and liveliness, along with solicitous suggestions for our welfare. During some discussion at the end of a session it came to light that every woman in the group was a mother and grandmother except for Celia, who reported that she 'had not been blessed with children', although she had tried to conceive for many years. Many of the women (and men) had as many as six or more children, and now had twenty or so grandchildren. For many, mothering seemed to be a totally natural role, and simply a matter of 'falling in love with each baby' as it arrived. I began to realize that childlessness must have been a very difficult thing to come to terms with for Celia, as child bearing and rearing was such a dominant pattern in the West Indian culture. Celia commented that it had been very hard for her to accept her loss, but that it had 'seemed to be God's will'. Celia had worked all her life as a nurse with children and had lots of contact with her nephews and nieces, so she had found positive ways of sublimating her capacity for mothering and parenting. As a woman from a West Indian cultural background Celia has had to face, in Erikson's terms, the adult challenge of generativity versus stagnation, without the possibility of biological reproduction as an option.

Marjorie

In noticing the individuality of each person's movement and personality in the group I began to let go of some of my stereotypical projections and racist assumptions. Not every woman was a large and solid Earth Goddess! From the outset there seemed to be something unusual about Marjorie. Sometimes her movements seemed to be very unco-ordinated and disconnected, with a split between the upper and lower halves of her body. Often her movements were stiff, with the sense that she was going through the motions physically, but with no connection to her inner self. Marjorie also seemed to be slightly embarrassed and confused when it was her turn to initiate a movement and share it with others. Following others' movements seemed to be acceptable for Marjorie, although I always had a sense of her withholding. Over the months this did not seem to change much, and on some level Marjorie remained an outsider within the group. On one occasion when I danced with Marjorie as a partner I sensed something scornful and dismissive on her part to do with the very act of dancing itself, as though she was being cajoled into doing something against her will. This part of Marjorie came out strongly one session when the issue of sexuality and morality came to the fore.

It was a hot summer's day when Betsy, a very gutsy lady in the group, came in wearing shorts and a skimpy top. I noticed a little snort of disapproval from Marjorie, who always wore tracksuit bottoms underneath her dress, whatever the weather. Betsy had a twinkle in her eye and asked me, whilst we were getting the room ready, whether I had 'got a bit of something last night with my boyfriend'. The impression one got from Betsy, from her speech and her movement, was that at 68 she was still very much interested in sex and, as she said, hoping to 'get plenty of it' when she joined her husband in Jamaica in a couple of months' time.

With the warm weather, few clothes on, and the influence of Betsy's remarks, the dancing during the session became very sexy with lots of pelvic movements that had a kind of daring quality, even though there were no men in the group at that time. Betsy started to do limbo dance movements, with everyone clapping, when Marjorie suddenly stopped dancing, sat down and shouted out 'I'm not doing that! It's not right, it's not Christian. My own mother would never let me do that.' It emerged as we talked about this that Marjorie had been brought up with a very strict form of Christian religious practice in which any physical expression of natural sexual feelings was forbidden. Marjorie had internalized these values and restrictions and lived by them all her life. Betsy challenged Marjorie by saying 'But your mother isn't here any more, so you don't have to do as she says. And anyway, it's good exercise for your body, doing all this. It helps my arthritis. I don't feel the pain so much.' Marjorie's religious convictions had been such a big part of her life, and patterns that, although she agreed to join in with movements like pelvic tilting and pelvic floor exercises, it would be for health reasons alone.

Marjorie got used to moving these parts of herself, but always remained slightly on guard, never dancing with abandon. During the last couple of years Marjorie has developed multiple physical problems such as diabetes, hypothyroidism, and Parkinson's disease which have handicapped her health, the last in particular having affected her ability to initiate functional movements such as feeding and dressing herself and walking. It is as though Marjorie's earlier movement patterns of rigidity and withholding hinted at how her later life might evolve. The symptoms of Parkinson's disease are muscular rigidity, tremor, and bradykinesia (difficulty in initiating a movement). Marjorie still comes to my sessions, but now attends a group more specifically for people who are housebound with disabilities.

CONCLUSIONS

My first conclusion, through thoroughly considering the position of older people in our society and current practice in dance movement therapy with this population, is that ageism has been very present in training provision and opportunities for dance movement therapy with elders. With the massive increase of older people living longer now and in the future, this group cannot afford to remain a disadvantaged minority living on the margins of life, for that is both a loss and a split in the whole of society and in ourselves. I regard the promotion of dance movement therapy with older people as a contribution towards a healing of this split and a remedying of this loss. We will all become old despite the present culture in which youth and glamour are idealized. Older people, along with other marginalized minorities in our society, need to be accepted and valued as worthwhile human beings with a valuable contribution to make.

Secondly, I would agree with some of the American practitioners that a focus on somatic issues is as important as a psychological focus for older people. Physical and psychological well-being are very much inseparable; we really are whole beings and it is only our thinking and attitudes which split mind and body into separate entities. Dance movement therapy can address the whole person and take into account individual differences between different generations of older people from a fit and newly retired 60-year-old to someone of 98 years who is now bed-ridden and can hardly move. Dance movement therapy can also include and validate the characteristics of different ethnic minorities' elders, and help to integrate this diversity and richness into our whole society.

Finally, dance movement therapy with older people must no longer be hidden in corners or kept under wraps. It is growing and coming to life in all sorts of venues and situations. It is an extremely valuable form of therapeutic work, not only for the older people themselves, but also for those therapists and teachers working with them. We need to let older people inform us, surprise us, and teach us of what they are truly capable, of how personal growth and development are possible at any age or stage of life.

SUMMARY

This chapter introduced the idea of a culture of ageing; how growing older in our society is affected by ageist attitudes which compound the physical and emotional losses of ill-health and bereavement. DMT provision can be affected by ageism in our our society and we need to be vigilant in combating this in our approach to our work in DMT in order to validate this population, whatever the culture and background.

NOTES

1 From a definition formulated by the Association of Dance Movement Therapy, c/o Arts Therapies Department, Springfield Hospital, Glenburnie Road, London SW17 7DJ.
2 The Feldenkrais method works for economy of movement with a minimum of muscular effort. The movements are done lying on the floor with gravity largely eliminated so that the neuro-muscular system is given the opportunity to change towards greater flexibility and co-ordination in movement. The method is outlined in greater detail in the book entitled *Awareness Through Movement* by Moshe Feldenkrais (1980) Harmondsworth, Middx: Penguin.

REFERENCES

Chaiklin, H. (ed.) (1975) *Marian Chace: Her Papers*, Columbia: American Dance Therapy Association.
Comfort, A. (1977) *A Good Age*, London: Mitchell Beazley.
Cumming, E. and Henry, W. E. (1961) *Growing Old: The Process of Disengagement*, New York: Basic Books.
Erikson, E. (1977) *Childhood and Society*, Herts: Triad Paladin.
Gardner, C. and Wethered, A. (1987), 'The therapeutic value of movement and dance', in L. Burr (ed.) *Therapy through Movement*, Nottingham: Nottingham Rehabilitation Press.
Garnet, E. D. (1974) 'A movement therapy for older people', in K. Mason (ed.) *Focus on Dance VII*, Reston, VA: American Alliance of Health, Physical Education and Recreation.

—— (1982) *Movement is Life: A Wholistic Approach to Exercise for Older Adults*, Princetown, NJ: Princetown Book Company.

Hendricks, J. and Hendricks, C. D. (1977) *Ageing in Mass Society*, Winthrop.

Keatinge, O. (1989) *Physical Recreation in Elderly People*, London Borough of Hackney.

Kelleman, S. (1985) *Emotional Anatomy*, Berkeley, CA: Centre Press.

Leventhal, M. (1988) 'The dance of life', unpublished article.

Lowe, G. (1976) *The Growth of Personality*, Harmondsworth, Middx: Penguin.

North, M. (1972) *Personality Assessment Through Movement*, London: Macdonald & Evans.

Pasch, J. (1982) *Movement for Old People*, Association of Dance Movement Therapy Publications, c/o Arts Therapies Department, Springfield Hospital, Glenburnie Road, London SW17 7DJ.

Salmon, P. (1985) *Living in Time*, London: Dent.

Sandel, S. L, and Read, D. (1987) *Waiting at the Gate: Creativity and Hope in the Nursing Home*, New York: Howarth Press.

Stanley, J. (ed.) (1989) *To Make Ends Meet*, Older Women's Project: Pensioners' Link, 17 Balfe St, London N1.

Ward, T. (1989) *New Age Against Ageism*, Search Project, 74 Adelaide Terrace, Newcastle on Tyne NE4 4BX.

Wethered, A. (1976) *Drama and Movement in Therapy*, Plymouth: Macdonald & Evans.

Chapter 5

Individual dance movement therapy in an in-patient psychiatric setting

Gayle Liebowitz

INTRODUCTION

In this chapter I propose to explore what dance movement therapy can offer to the treatment of psychosis, firstly, through a discussion of theory and, secondly, through recounting the case of a schizophrenic woman. In addition, I will also take a look at how staff dynamics within an institutional setting can affect the DMT treatment process.

A psychiatric hospital caters for individuals who need an environment where they can recover from severe disturbance, usually a psychotic illness. The aetiology and treatment of psychosis have long been debated and the theories include such contenders as the biochemical, genetic, psychological, and social/environmental, though as yet there has been no conclusive evidence proving any one theory in particular. In this chapter I will emphasize the environmental model which supports the hypothesis that difficulty in the early pre-verbal mother–child relationship is a determining factor in the development of psychosis. I am proposing that dance movement therapy, which provides an opportunity to explore the relationship of self to others through bodily movement, is a valuable treatment of choice for this patient population.

Theory

The philosophical underpinnings of my work combine existentialism and psychic determinism. I have attempted for years to reconcile the apparent conflict between these two orientations. Both approaches have served to offer me something: psychic determinism, how the past influences the present, and existentialism, a subjective experience of ontology. Psychiatrist Murray Cox writes eloquently of the harmony of these opposites,

> Psychic determinism may have led the patient to the brink of the disclosure, so that the material which has hitherto been unconscious

is about to enter consciousness. . . . It is as though the existential component is a kind of emotional range-finder, which indicates that the dynamics of formulation based on psychic determinism is 'on target', so that the patient responds to an intervention by feeling 'how true' rather than 'how dare you'.

(Cox 1978: 112)

Existentialism is a science of being. It concerns itself not only with objective experience but also subjective experience, not only what is 'abstractly true' but what is 'existentially real' for the living person (May 1958: 13). Existential psychiatrist Rollo May has stressed that we must study not only an individual's experience but the individual who is doing the experiencing (May 1958: 14), or, as Tillich expresses it, 'with the accent on the inner personal character of man's immediate experience' (Tillich 1944: 44). Existential psychotherapists strive to elucidate the existential reality of the patient through a process of *being with* rather than through a process of intellectually analysing. According to existential writers the body has a central place in human existence. In fact, existential psychiatrist Medard Boss contends that 'Human bodyhood is the bodying forth of ways of being in which we are dwelling and which constitute our existence at any given moment' (Boss 1979: 102). DMT aims to explore the patient's existence through bodily movement. In dance movement therapy a meeting occurs between the therapist's and the patient's qualities of movement, posture, gesture, rhythm, and phrasing. Merleau-Ponty, philosopher, states, 'It is through my body that I understand other people and it is through my body that I perceive things' (Merleau-Ponty 1962: 186). Through moving with the patient and stepping into the patient's movement patterns the dance movement therapist can experience first hand what it is like to be the patient and in so doing can achieve an instantaneous empathic awareness.

Within this *meeting* between therapist and client the body speaks not only in the immediacy of the moment but also in the past. Memories of past bodily meetings continuously influence bodily expression in the present. Psychoanalysis contributes to our understanding of this bodily past. Freud theorized in his early writings that 'the ego was first and foremost a body ego' (Freud 1923: 26). The ego, one's sense of self, the conscious link with the external world, begins with a world of sensations; internal rumblings of physiological processes and external stimulations of the environment including visual, olfactory, auditory, and tactile. These physical experiences become the rudimentary beginnings of the ego. The infant's self has no demarcating boundaries but rather is an extension of the mother's body; internal and external are interchangeable. The developing infant begins to discriminate between their body and that of the mother and eventually, if all goes well, a sense of separateness and individuation is achieved (Mahler 1968). Psychoanalytical literature suggests that psychotic individuals have been hindered in their psychological growth by environmental and also possibly constitutional deficiencies and thus have not been able to establish a secure sense of themselves (Fairbairn 1941; Klein 1946; Bowlby 1957; Winnicott 1960; Balint 1968; Mahler 1968). Winnicott (1960, 1962) emphasized the importance of 'good enough' mothering which consists of the mother meeting her infant's physical and emotional needs. Through internalizing this good enough mothering the infant begins to build up a 'continuity of being', moving from an unintegrated ego state to an integrated one. When this continuity of being is interrupted by inadequate or inconsistent care, it gives rise to 'unthinkable anxiety'. Winnicott states that 'such interruptions constitute annihilation and are evidently associated with pain of psychotic quality and intensity' (Winnicott 1960: 52).

DMT, which concerns itself with bodily relationships, has the ability to connect with past bodily memories in order to work through these primitive body experiences. Psychoanalytic psychotherapist and movement therapist Dosamantes-Alperson writes, 'Since our earliest relationships are primarily transacted through motoric and imagistic modes, what recollections we may have of them, may only be available to us in the form of bodily sensations, movements, and images' (Dosamantes-Alperson 1987: 6).

How are these memories stored in the body? Wilhelm Reich, early follower of Freud, suggested that emotions were repressed in the body in the form of muscular tension or character armouring (Reich 1945). Reich believed that, by massaging muscles and releasing tension, the therapist would also release feelings that had been frozen in the body. This freezing is often noticeable in the rigid and bound body posture and movement of the psychotic individual, indicating a defence against feelings. Psychoanalyst, Judith Kestenberg (1975) has related Anna Freud's psychosexual stages (1936) to developmental movement patterns. Kestenberg introduced the idea that 'motor apparati are put in the service of developing mental structures' (Kestenberg 1975: 189); that each developmental stage brings with it phase-specific tasks to master and corresponding emotional issues that will need to be worked through. For example, a child who learns to walk and use his weight in the vertical plane can now physically move away from the mother and will begin to deal with the issue of separation. When individuals have not adequately worked through a stage they will tend to regress and fixate to this point during the therapeutic process, expressing issues particular to this phase of development. In dance movement therapy this regression occurs on a body level, the repertoire of movement patients bring to the session revealing their personal developmental histories. Movement qualities and rhythms from stages not yet integrated into the personality will either be lacking or will predominate, presenting themselves to be repeated and worked through in the therapy session.

As psychotic individuals have experienced trauma very early in life their movement profiles reflect patterns that have not progressed beyond the oral phase, revealing unclear and diffuse spatial patterns (lack of an awareness of direction in space), minimum weight efforts (no sense of body weight or of having the feet on the ground), unusually slow or quick timing, extremes of flow (very bound and tense musculature and movements or free, continuous, and uncontained movements), segmentation (pauses between phrases of movement), fragmentation (one body part moving out of synchrony with another), and bizarre gestures and postures (Davis 1970; Dell 1970; North 1972). In general, there is a widespread restriction of the movement repertoire, a lack of spontaneous movement, and difficulties in relating to others on a movement level, including under- or over-attunement, fear of physical touch, or a disregard for body boundaries (Fisher and Cleveland 1965). It is worth pointing out that development, even with psychotic patients, may sometimes be patchy and a more advanced stage may be mastered before an earlier one. This will mean, however, that the foundations upon which these higher level skills rest are tenuous and may deteriorate quickly under stress. It has also been questionable as to whether the administration of psychotropic drugs (major tranquillizers) has affected the movement profiles of hospitalized patients. Research has provided preliminary evidence to the contrary, suggesting that movement patterns are not drastically altered, though motility may be somewhat reduced due to the sedating qualities of the drugs (Cardone and Olson 1969; Davis 1970).

TECHNIQUES

The description of the psychotic movement profile does appear to reflect a continuity of being that has been interrupted and inconsistent and leads us to believe that psychotic individuals may also have a view of their bodies as undeveloped and unreliable. One's personal perception of one's body, including images, feelings, and phantasies, make up one's *body image*. Paul Schilder (1950), psychoanalyst, who has done extensive research on the body image concept believes that one's body image is related to one's sense of self. Whereas a realistic body image will reflect a firm sense of identity, Schilder postulated that distorted body images were reflections of disturbed psychological states, that 'mental suffering finds its way into somatic expression' (Schilder 1950: 301). Schilder was also the first to note that movement loosens the body image, 'and leads from a change in the body image to a change in the psychic attitude' (Schilder 1950: 208).

German psychiatrist and psychoanalyst Gisela Pankow (1961, 1981) suggests that psychotic individuals have 'a dissociated image' of their bodies and a perception of their bodies as fragmented, in parts rather than as a whole. In a method she calls 'dynamic structurization', Pankow works towards helping the psychotic integrate a realistic body image. Reading Pankow one has the impression that she is a pioneer in dance movement therapy; however, she diverges in that she focuses on sculpting clay images and therefore works outside the body. In dance movement therapy, integration takes place within the body, through working with the body, and in relation to another body (patient and therapist). When working with psychotics we encourage body awareness by, for example, circling and shaking body parts, mark body boundaries by tapping and patting legs, arms, and torso, and encourage connections to be felt between one body part and another through stretching. Interaction with others begins through, for example, pulling, pushing, clapping, swinging, and rocking. Props, such as balls, hoops, stretch clothes, mirrors, and cushions, are used to encounter the environment and make an impact on the world. Developmentally we are working at a very early level, a pre-verbal, pre-oedipal stage when infants have not yet separated from their mothers and are still discovering their bodies and learning about themselves through exploration.

Recreating motility during this phase is not enough but must take place in the presence of another person, the therapist. There is not only a real existential relationship between therapist and patient but, we also know from psychoanalysis, there is a transference relationship. Transference, as defined by Sandler, is:

> a specific illusion which develops in regard to the other person, which, unbeknown to the subject, represents, in some of its features, a repetition of a relationship towards an important figure in the person's past.
>
> (Sandler et al. 1973: 49)

Freud originally stated that persons with 'narcissistic neurosis' (psychotics) had no capacity for developing transference (Freud 1917: 447). None the less, later analysts argued that this was not necessarily true. Rather than manifesting a transference neurosis it has been posited that psychotic individuals engage in a 'transference psychosis' (Rosenfeld 1971, 1987), or, as Margaret Little calls it, a 'delusional transference' (Little 1986). By this she means that psychotic individuals respond to therapists not *as if* they were the mother-father but are the mother-father. Psychotic individuals perceive the therapist not as a separate person but as a part of themselves, similar to the infant who is fused in symbiosis with the mother. Thus the psychotic exists in a non-differentiated state and has difficulty distinguishing the *me* from the *not me*. In dance movement therapy the 'delusional transference' becomes the *delusional body transference*, a repertoire of movements that the psychotic exhibits in the presence of the therapist which is identical to movement patterns that had been exhibited to a significant figure in the past. The dance movement therapist's personal movement response to the patient, which reflects the therapist's unresolved issues with persons from the past, is called the therapist's *body counter-transference*. An example of this process is when dance movement therapists become aware that they have continued to move with an oral libidinal rhythm which promotes attachment (Kestenberg 1975) when a client has previously introduced an oral sadistic rhythm which promotes separation (Kestenberg 1975). In this case, the therapists have hindered the client's early strivings towards separation and it indicates that the therapists have not sufficiently worked through this issue themselves. In addition, through projective identification, therapists will pick up movement qualities and rhythms from the patient and reproduce them in their bodies. These acquired patterns acquaint the therapist with the psychotic's simmering emotional life and therefore it is paramount that the therapist recognize and distinguish the origins of these movement patterns from the body counter-transference. As much as possible, the therapist must sustain an awareness of these bodily responses during the session. However, when there is an impediment to this awareness, the supervisory session offers the therapist a space to reflect on and clarify the therapeutic process. The potency of feelings that may arise when working with a psychotic population indicates that personal therapy is an imperative prerequisite.

Margaret Little asserts that 'the giving up of the delusion starts from the discovery of the body moving in response to an urge and finding contact' (Little 1986: 85). Movements that arise from the patient must be acknowledged either verbally, or even concretely, through touch. These movements, Little continues, are 'assertions of the self and a starting point for developing relationships' (1986: 98). These statements are reminiscent of the early mother–child relationship when the mother acts as both mirror and feedback system for her infant (Brazelton *et al.* 1974). Likewise, as the mother functions as an ego support by organizing and giving meaning to her infant's responses, in a similar manner the dance movement therapist responds to the psychotic patient by making verbal and non-verbal interventions.

The constructiveness of verbal interpretation when working with psychotic patients has been a controversial subject amongst analysts. Balint (1968), in particular, has stressed the pointlessness of words when working at a pre-verbal level, a level where symbolic thought has not yet evolved because internalization of the primary object has not been achieved.

> Words become, in fact, unreliable and unpredictable. . . . the ana-
> lyst's task is to understand what lies behind the patient's words;
> the problem is only how to communicate this understanding to a
> regressed patient.

> (Balint 1968: 175, 177)

Balint advises staying with the patient in silence with the aim of communicating understanding. Here, I would like to suggest that the dance movement therapist has the skills to work within this *silent understanding* by responding to the client's non-verbal expression. For the dance movement therapist this means tuning in to and reflecting the patient's movement qualities, rhythms, and phrasing which may be as minimal as a foot tapping, a breathing rhythm, a hand gesture, or the nod of the head. In this way, the dance movement therapists meet the client's gesture with a gesture of their own, one that communicates a quality of *being with*, a response that will be acceptable to the patient and will ultimately strengthen the therapeutic alliance. Morever, dance movement therapists have the advantage in that not only can they communicate benevolent understanding, but they can also interpret on a level that is accessible to the psychotic.

Due to the psychotic's deficient capacity for symbolization, there is a tendency for the psychotic to think concretely and thus movement is perceived literally – as a physical movement of muscles and joints, as a rendition of an actual activity, or as a personal idiosyncratic 'symbolic equation' (Segal 1955). For example, the circling of a hand may be simply seen as a movement of the hand joints and muscles in a circular direction, or as an imitation of twirling a firework, or the hand may be experienced as having the powerful force of a firework. In contrast, a metaphorical understanding of this movement might be as an expression of one's aggressive feelings which are feared to be dangerously explosive. A verbal interpretation based on this latter formulation may baffle or threaten a psychotic patient. Instead, the dance movement therapist has the option of responding to the patient's communication in various ways: a) by reflecting the movement the therapist acknowledges the patient's feelings; b) by expanding the movement the therapist draws attention to the patient's potentiality; c) by diminishing the movement the therapist offers the possibility of containing the feelings expressed; d) by accentuating a movement the therapist emphasizes one aspect that may be particularly important; and e) by contrasting the movement the therapist proposes alternative ways of being that may be more adaptive.

I do believe that at a later stage in our work with psychotic people these non-verbal interpretations will need to be made verbal and it is at this point that words are necessary. We must remember that words are part of the totality of the mother's care for her infant. Words make sounds which have audible rhythm and cadence and can soothe or irritate. In so much as therapists' verbal utterances are in synchrony with their body movement, then they will communicate a quality of feeling. Rosenfeld (1987) speaks about words taking on a holding function within the therapy session. He insists that, by using words, the therapist acknowledges that patients are still adults and does not infantilize them. Words also link primary process to secondary process thought and by using words as well as movement the therapist facilitates the evolution towards symbolization within the context of the movement relationship.

A major part of the process of interpretation in therapy includes the elucidation of the patient's defence mechanisms. Spotnitz (1985) proposes that schizophrenia, in itself, is a defence against the expression of aggressive impulses which are mobilized in response to a frustrating environment, but are then suppressed in fear of rejection or retaliation.

In an effort to eliminate bad feelings the psychotic may project them into the therapist, not only to be rid of them, but so that they may be contained by the therapist. The patient may now attack the bad parts of themselves vicariously through the therapist (Klein 1946). One of the goals of therapy with the psychotic individual is to restore these bad parts to their rightful owner, namely, the patient. In the therapist's attempts to do so, the patient may experience the therapist as persecutory, for the psychotic believes that it is now the therapist that is making them feel bad. The flood of feelings that can arise is so intense that the psychotic may fear becoming overwhelmed. In dance movement therapy this may manifest itself in the patient becoming very resistant to moving for fear of unleashing a multitude of feelings. This means that the therapist must follow the patient's lead, gradually modulating the extent and range of movement within the session, so that patients do not become threatened by their own movement impulses. This is especially important because many psychotic patients have poor impulse control and cannot self-regulate and thus the potential for *acting out* is a reality.

Freud (1914) originally defined *acting out* as an unconsciously motivated behaviour that expresses aspects of one's relationship to past significant others and which is enacted through action (both inside and outside the therapy session) instead of being remembered through verbal discourse. Transference can be considered a form of acting out within the session that facilitates the therapeutic process (for example, yelling at one's therapist when one is really angry at one's parents) whereas acting out that occurs outside the session (such as becoming angry at one's boss rather than at one's therapist) can be detrimental to the therapeutic process. Verbal psychotherapists often fear that DMT, which is primarily an action therapy, may promote acting out. Cognitive thought processes have not yet replaced motoric discharge in the psychotic, and so, through a process called somatization, affects are often expressed by a physical response. However, it is worth remembering that the *raison d'être* for employing movement is explicitly in order to connect up with bodily memories and the feelings associated with them. Therefore, unlike in verbal psychotherapy, movement, rather than talking, becomes the method of remembering and expression. It is when movement becomes a *re-enactment* of an experience from the past with significant others, as opposed to moving *about* an experience, that it can be deemed acting out, for example, pretending to take a bath is different from actually taking a bath (see case illustration).

As previously stated, psychotic individuals cannot always differentiate between the therapist and past significant others, and, therefore, acting out is difficult to prevent. Balint (1968) believes that a certain amount of acting out must be tolerated when working with regressed individuals. What must not be tolerated however is physical violence or sexually disinhibited behaviour which is not appropriate in the context of the therapy session. The therapy session must be safe enough for individuals to express themselves through their physical bodies without the fear of going out of control. The dance movement therapist may therefore need to defuse a build-up of motor impulses through redirection or channelling of one movement quality into another (for example, a punching movement may be redirected to the floor rather than at someone or a quick swing may be slowed down), through restrictions of spatial boundaries (confining the movement to a smaller area of space), or, even, actual physical restraint of the patient's body.

Physical contact within the psychoanalytic session is traditionally anathema, though several independent analysts have explored the possibility of allowing physical touch when working with very regressed patients (Little 1986; Casement 1982). The decision whether to touch or not in dance movement therapy depends on the meaning that is attributed to the physical contact by the patient. To the psychotic client, touch is very much an expression of early infantile gratification. For some, touch is sought after in order to get physically close to the point of phantasized merging with the therapist, whilst for others touch is experienced as a seduction and intrusion. In general, touch must always be used with discretion, for though it may enhance the transferential relationship in one case, it may contaminate the relationship in another.

This has been a summary of those issues I believe are important to be aware of when working in DMT with a psychotic population. In the next section, to demonstrate the application of theory to practice, I present the case of a young woman diagnosed as chronic schizophrenic.

CASE ILLUSTRATION

The ward to which I was assigned had recently been changed from an acute ward to a rehabilitation ward accommodating primarily chronic schizophrenics. This is a group of patients who cannot survive alone outside the hospital setting and need to live in a supportive environment. Unfortunately, there is currently a shortage of sheltered group homes in the community and therefore, to address this problem, hospital managements have created long-stay rehabilitation units within the hospital.

My reception was not what one would call hospitable, from the patients' side that is. I was scowled at, shouted at, told to f . . . off, and then ignored. This reaction to a new face is a common phenomenon when working with chronic schizophrenics as their fears of being intruded upon are primary and for protection they shield themselves with hostility, indifference, and withdrawal. Sometimes though, one is approached with interest and that first morning in April I was greeted by an overweight West Indian woman in her mid-20s wearing tight blue jeans, a jersey top that didn't quite reach below her navel, and a bandana around her head. She surprised me by asking if we could talk and so I set up a meeting that afternoon.

Suzanne first came to the attention of psychiatric services when she was 22 and found to be living in squalid conditions, pregnant with a second child. She was treated on an out-patient basis with anti-psychotic medication, and with support from the community psychiatric nurse appeared to improve. Two years later, however, Suzanne relapsed after defaulting on her medication. She was admitted to hospital and soon after was placed on the rehabilitation ward. A year and a half later, at the time when I arrived, Suzanne was still on this ward.

Suzanne spent our first session telling me about her life between puffs of a cigarette. She expressed interest in continuing with the sessions especially as she perceived them as being able to help her lose weight and so we scheduled a meeting the following week.

Suzanne arrived the next week looking distinctly uncomfortable. 'I've never done this before', she stated shyly, displaying a mixture of fear and ambivalence as compared to the previous week's brashness. She twiddled her thumbs and when I pointed this out to her she said that she felt nervous. I initiated a simple movement warm-up so that I could make an assessment of her movement repertoire. She followed me compliantly. Her free flow (unrestrained) movement in the pelvic region and her continuous talk about her sexual escapades led me to suspect that she had difficulty in the area of sexuality. In fact, as her movement repertoire was restricted and reflected an early developmental level, I hypothesized that she could not engage in mature sexual intimacy but used sex as a way to fulfil her infantile dependency needs.

In our third session I began by suggesting warm-up exercises for each body part. Within a few minutes Suzanne had backed up against the wall with her hands behind her back and then abruptly sat down. She said she was going to leave the session because she did not like her body and asked if people could have operations to alter how they looked. It seemed as if the movement had called forth negative feelings about her self that were so painful that Suzanne wanted to get away from the room immediately. Suzanne then stated that her mother had fairer skin than hers and had beat her up and lied to her. I wondered if she was really referring to me in her statement. After all, I had fair skin (white) and I had suggested movements that had the effect of making her feel bad. Though it appeared that Suzanne was projecting feelings about her mother I had actually become the nasty, fair-skinned mother in the delusional body transference.

In these initial sessions Suzanne was extremely passive and resistant. I continued to introduce structured movement warm-ups consisting of flexing, stretching, and shaking body parts in the hope that the movement would make contact with her on a pre-verbal level. Suzanne would sit, unresponsive, with eyes glazed and unfocused, staring in front of her, her body rigid, defending against my approach. She would mechanically follow my movements until suddenly she would find a movement amusing, or, as she described it, unusual. She would then begin to giggle and this would break the awkward, tense silence between us. This transition period, as I came to perceive it, revealed the magnitude of the void that Suzanne had to bridge between one session and the next. Unfortunately, the sessions could only be once a week and so the separation appeared as a break in the continuity of our relationship. In each session we had to begin again the process of establishing a link.

I was not sure how to penetrate Suzanne's defensive posture until Suzanne herself provided me with an opportunity. I was writing up my notes in the nurses' office immediately after one session when I caught sight of Suzanne through the window. She was dancing provocatively, wiggling her hips and laughing with another patient. The session we had just ended had been unproductive and resistant with Suzanne moving hesitantly with bound flow. Here she was, though, dancing with spontaneity and free flow, in clear view of me but acting out of the session time. I mentioned this incident to Suzanne the following week and indicated that her dancing had looked like it belonged inside the session. She nodded her head saying nothing; however, she began to show this other side of herself within the session.

Soon, the interchange between talking and moving became a noticeable feature of the sessions with Suzanne. She would arrive at a session and talk continuously until an anxiety-provoking issue was raised when she would then request to move. Or vice versa, she would be dancing when a movement would trigger a thought, feeling, or memory and Suzanne would sit down and begin to talk. Though it appeared that relevant issues were being avoided by engaging in the opposite mode, and indeed sometimes they were, on another level Suzanne had discovered a method of self-regulation. When movement became too direct and raw then she would distance herself through verbalization. When words became too disturbing and incomprehensible she would switch to an action form which allowed her expression and tension discharge.

I had managed to obtain the use of a room at the day hospital for Suzanne's therapy session instead of the tiny room we had used on the ward. It was larger, carpeted, and had a window, piano, and mirror. This mirror was to become an essential ingredient in the process of therapy. In the beginning, middle, and end of each session Suzanne would ritualistically look into the mirror and remark on how she thought she looked. One day Suzanne suddenly became aware of me reflecting her movement in the mirror and exclaimed that I was imitating her. I asked Suzanne if she would prefer me to sit down and watch. 'Yes', she replied, 'I have to get used to myself'. I began to realize that Suzanne's repeated checking in the mirror was her way of confirming her existence and was an attempt to integrate a coherent sense of self (Lacan 1977). However, her body image was inconsistent and sometimes she would look 'fat' and 'ugly' and at other times she would look 'all right' and 'pretty'. Suzanne's perception of herself at any given moment was often a reflection of her transference relationship with me. When she was angry at the beginning of a session, then her face looked 'darker', but by the end of a session, after this anger had been expressed, she would feel 'lighter'. In a sense, I also acted as a mirror, reflecting her self back to her in a palatable form, and as her harsh internal objects became modified in her relationship to me, her body image was also transformed.

One morning a week I ran a dance movement therapy group on Suzanne's ward. Occasionally she would participate but more often than not she would remain for a few minutes and then leave. One day a patient pretended to take a bath in the group session. Suzanne had been watching but did not join in. Later in her individual session Suzanne suggested taking a bath. She mimed the entire procedure from turning the tap on, washing body parts, drying off, and dressing. As the therapist-mother it was important for me to be present during this symbolic bath ritual and to acknowledge Suzanne's bodily needs. On the ward Suzanne would absolutely refuse to bathe but in the safe space of the therapy session Suzanne could care for her body.

The bath session marked the end of the initial phase of our relationship. Suzanne now became actively resistant and angry. The conflict that precipitated this anger was my refusal to accompany her to the hospital cashier to obtain her money during session time. She begged the nurses to take her but they were adamant that she must go to her session. She pleaded with me but to no avail. Suzanne was furious. She missed one session and went to visit her mother. She screamed at me the following week, 'You don't own me. My mum comes first. I'm never coming to your session again!' Suzanne could not yet perceive the session as valuable to herself and began to engage splitting processes. I became the devouring bad mother forcing her into a witches' gingerbread house and her real mother became all good. I didn't see her that day but, interestingly enough, I heard from the nursing staff that she had taken a bath instead.

Nevertheless, Suzanne did return and in the next few weeks her persecutory self made its appearance within the movement sessions. Now when she stopped abruptly during a dance she would venture to explain what disturbing feelings had arisen. Rotating her hips brought up fears of homosexuality and she worried that people would call her a lesbian. She would distort my words and accuse me of calling her names and I would have to reassure her to prevent her from walking out. She projected feelings of inadequacy about herself onto me, as when she told me that I looked like an elephant and then, apprehensive that I might cast the insult back, she berated me for mocking her. This hostile attitude continued over the next few months with a recurring scenario of Suzanne refusing to attend the therapy sessions and yelling aggressively that she did not like me. Eventually she would calm down and decide to attend a session though she would defiantly announce that she wasn't going to do anything. Once in the therapy room however, Suzanne would look in the mirror and each week she would comment on a part of her body and compare herself with me. Yet, in spite of all her challenging behaviour, Suzanne choreographed a dance with me which she based on movement sequences she had learned in dance classes during her school days. This dance displayed a wider range of movement, consisting of skips, turns, rolls on the floor, and jumps. She even dared to make contact by clapping my hands as part of this dance.

At other times though Suzanne would refuse to move. She would keep me at a distance by placing herself on the opposite side of the room and specifying that she did not want to touch or sit near me. I would then join in her resistance, waiting for her to take the initiative. Eventually, Suzanne revealed what was at the heart of her resistance when she admitted that she was afraid of going mad. It seemed that as Suzanne became more attached to me and got in touch with her feelings through movement, she began to fear losing control of herself and becoming overwhelmed by unconscious impulses.

Gradually, Suzanne began to disclose more about her inner world. She told me that when she was at school the other girls had called her 'blackie' and to lighten her skin she had attempted to bleach her face. She was convinced that the cream she had used at the age of twelve had burned her face for life. She knew in reality that her face bore no physical scars but her concern was evidence of an internal perception of herself as a scarred individual. In the formation of a bodily ego/self the skin forms a boundary (Bick 1968) and in Suzanne's case this boundary had not been firmly established. Hence, the burning of skin represented an erosion of body boundaries resulting in a distorted body image.

Death was also an issue that concerned and worried Suzanne. When I asked her what movement she would like to finish with at the end of a session she enquired whether I thought she was dying, the imminent separation being experienced as an annihilation of self. Breathing exercises also confronted Suzanne with her existence and the possibility of no breath at all. Her sense of self was so elusive that her very existence was always in question.

On the ward Suzanne was a management problem. She was abusive to staff and refused to follow the ward programme. She smoked in bed, would not wash, and was sexually provocative to other patients. The nurses grew more impatient and angry, arguments ensued and when Suzanne yelled, they yelled back. Suzanne became the impossible patient, the type of patient that made their job so despairing and frustrating.

One night Suzanne punched and kicked a female nurse. The psychiatrist reprimanded her and threatened her with police action and imprisonment. Suzanne responded to this with flippancy and showed no remorse. She said it was the nurse who had started the fight by calling her names, and, besides, she did not care if she went to prison. Suzanne had acted out and displaced her anger and envy of me onto another female figure in the hospital structure. Soon after this incident, the ward decided that they could not cope with Suzanne and made the decision to transfer her to an acute ward where she would then be discharged. Indeed, Suzanne was being pawned off by one authority to another. Unfortunately, it seemed as if the staff had become enmeshed in a 'dramatization' (Hinshelwood 1987: 23) of counter-transference feelings. The ward staff had projected all that was bad on the ward into Suzanne and now they were attempting to dispose of her. Thus, not only was Suzanne hopeless and despairing at this stage in the therapy, but the ward staff were hopeless and despairing, and I had become hopeless and despairing as well.

It was now August and my holiday was scheduled for September. I had prepared Suzanne for my departure earlier in the month and she had responded with 'Good, I'll be glad to be rid of you.' The last two sessions she refused to attend. When I did see her again in October, she still had not been transferred. Though she greeted my return with a big smile she punished me by not turning up for the first session. A new phase however was ushered in. Suzanne became totally dependent on me to the extent that she would wait outside the office until it was time for the session to begin. She became attached to a specific cassette tape of music that she would listen to over and over again, recorder on her lap, rocking side to side in a symbiotic oral rhythm (Kestenberg 1975).

Without warning I was informed that the funding for my post had been cut and that I would have to leave at the end of December. At the same time the ward staff lost all patience with Suzanne and made the decision to discharge her to a bed and breakfast. So fate had it that we would both be leaving. Suzanne was distraught and rocked herself in comfort, speaking about her fear of living alone and seeing ghosts. My announcement added to her misery, 'that's bad', she wailed. 'Who will I tell my problems to?' She stood up and performed a sad dance that ended with a prayer gesture, praying that she would get better.

Suzanne was convinced that she would be gone by the next day, insisting that her key worker had told her this, but, though I rang around the hospital, I could not confirm a discharge date. I felt irate! How could communication be so poor and a patient treated so inconsiderately? My anger was intensified by my own feelings of upset about the loss of my DMT post at the hospital. As she wiped away tears from her eyes Suzanne pleaded for advice, asserting that I was the only one she trusted. I could only offer out-patient sessions to her and hope that she would find her way back for them. As it turned out, Suzanne did show up the following week as there had been no available bed and breakfast.

The goals of the session now had to change to focus on our impending separation. Suzanne continued rocking to her favourite tape but she was angry and sullen. She regressed to a passive dependent attitude similar to our initial sessions eight months ago. She entreated me to tell her what to do. She accused me of 'mucking around' (the expression Suzanne used to indicate that one wasn't getting down to work) and making her feel bad, even suicidal. But then one day she had a thought, if I was leaving then perhaps we had better spend time talking. For the last three weeks then Suzanne resisted moving or dancing. This is not an uncommon phenomenon. As individuals approach separation they need to withdraw cathexis and to obtain an emotional distance which the verbal mode provides. I now suggested that we make a *goodbye book*, a tangible record of Suzanne's experience in therapy and a concrete representation of our relationship. Suzanne traced around her hands with a pen on the cover page and on the inside she traced around her special tape and wrote, 'I like movement; we use every part of the body'. She described her problems which consisted of a list of her body parts, and then sadly at the end of the list she wrote, 'all of me'. She drew a face in red ink explaining that it represented fire (her burnt face, I presumed) and commented that she wasn't pretty like the picture. I drew stick figures of her and me dancing together and wrote our names underneath. Suzanne then drew in my hair and earrings but no clothes and giggled at the idea of me being naked. At the end of the session Suzanne said that she was going to miss me and that she might cry.

In our final meeting together Suzanne announced that she was not going to write in the book and instead put on her favourite tape. After about twenty minutes of fast forwarding from song to song she commented that she had been 'mucking around'. She dedicated a song to me and walked over to the mirror remarking that she looked all right. She then asked me if I had bought her a Christmas gift. Over the past few weeks Suzanne had been pursuing the subject of Christmas gifts with me. I do not, generally, give gifts to patients but as our therapeutic process was going to be interrupted I had, after long deliberation, decided to make Suzanne a tape of her favourite songs so that she would, metaphorically speaking, take a good holding experience away with her. In retrospect, I questioned my motives for giving Suzanne a gift. I wondered if I had felt guilty about letting her down and had needed to compensate by giving her something in place of the missed sessions. I became aware of the effect of the gift the following week when Suzanne showed up for the group session, lunged forward to hug and kiss me, and announced that she fancied me. Since I had gratified one of her desires by giving her a gift, Suzanne now expected me to fulfil others. Knowing of Suzanne's confusion over sexuality, and the fact that she had kept my stick figure in the goodbye book naked, I should have been prepared for her response, but I wasn't. Instead I reacted out of anxiety by promptly pushing her away from me. I then realized that Suzanne had wanted to get close to me as an infant searches for the warmth of the mother's body. Unfortunately, Suzanne's only way of doing so was to act out sexually. Though this could not be worked through in the group, Suzanne's behaviour did stimulate a discussion about different types of relationships.

Before I left the ward Suzanne told me that the tape had been destroyed by another patient. I felt sad. Suzanne could not care for the tape any more than she could care for herself. As she was telling me this an elderly patient came up to me and shook my hand. Suzanne watched with interest and then solemnly offered her hand to me. We shook hands and said goodbye.

CONCLUSIONS

Let us now return to our original question: how does dance movement therapy contribute to the treatment of psychosis and how does the institutional setting influence this process? It is obvious that a major hindrance to the progression of Suzanne's therapy was the premature termination enforced by the hospital management, firstly, in financial cutbacks to the hospital budget and, secondly, on another level, as a consequence of the psychological group processes of the ward staff. This is, however, the reality of working within an institutional setting. Budgets are always a practical issue and as dance movement therapy is a newcomer to the hospital team it is often the first profession to be expendable.

Unfortunately, there is no way of getting around the powerful emotions that are projected from patients to staff (and vice versa) and often acted out to the detriment of the unit. This process is graphically illustrated in Suzanne's case, with staff becoming so entangled in Suzanne's angry feelings that they end up threatening her with transfer and discharge. Another problem that may arise is the sabotage by staff members of one's work out of envy that the dance movement therapist is able to establish a good rapport with a difficult patient. There may also be concerns that the therapy may stir up feelings that will make the patient worse. In the latter case, it is important for the therapist to explain that exploring feelings within the dance movement therapy session can actually contain rather than exacerbate distressing feelings, and, therefore, deter acting out rather than contributing to it. To prevent these factors from interfering with one's therapeutic work it is vital to maintain good relations with the rest of the staff through feedback sessions, written reports, and attendance at team meetings. Staff can also benefit from hearing the therapist's views and may even change their attitude and the manner in which they relate to patients. The dance movement therapist must not only support the staff but at the same time preserve the integrity of the therapeutic work. This balance at times requires a diplomatic service. It is however worthwhile to keep in mind, that, in as much as the institution can disrupt the therapeutic process, it can also serve as a holding environment, a place where psychotic individuals can be safe and protected until such time as they can be on their own. And, in a way, the hospital also supports the dance movement therapist, for the therapist can be assured that when the session is over the patient will be looked after and this is essential when working with regressed individuals.

Thus we have the paradox of the psychiatric hospital. On the one hand, it is bureaucratic, rigid, and impersonal, yet on the other hand it offers security, protection, and asylum. It aims to facilitate independence but a by-product of institutionalism is dependence. This paradox also reflects the ambivalence of many psychotic patients. Let us recall that Suzanne was extremely uncertain about leaving the hospital setting even though she complained about the nursing staff and admitted that she was becoming lazy. The idea of living in the community filled her with terror and she expressed concern about what people might think of her. Clearly, Suzanne's difficulty separating from the mother institution is mirrored in her struggle to differentiate from the symbiotic mother relationship with her own mother and with the therapist-mother in the delusional body transference.

Having placed Suzanne within this context let us now turn to the actual therapeutic work. In this chapter I have proposed that dance movement therapy is a valuable and beneficial treatment of choice with psychotic individuals because of the ability of movement to connect with early infantile body experiences. In the holding space of therapy patients are able to re-integrate a body image, stabilize body boundaries, and begin to differentiate themselves as a separate self from the other. When I asked Suzanne what contributed to her reversal in attitude from utter refusal to attend sessions to her utter devotion, she replied that the change occured when she realized that she could play a tape if she wished during the session. When Suzanne discovered that she could do as she liked, that she could *own* herself rather than being *owned* (controlled) by the mother-therapist, when she could, in her words, 'get used to herself', then the therapy became meaningful.

And it was through the discovery of her body that meaning was found. What the verbal could no longer express Suzanne expressed through bodily rhythms. The dance movement therapist was able to enter into this realm of rhythmic sensation derived from the past and maintain a link with the present, and it was just this link that brought Suzanne into relation with the mother-therapist, the *other* in the external world. The dance movement therapist holds, both physically and emotionally, the psychotic's body self together until such time as these individuals can hold their own body self together through internalization of the maternal object.

In conclusion, let us return to the existential moment in dance movement therapy. This is the moment that movement speaks of an individual's truth. The moment Suzanne's breath became the experience of non-breath, the moment Suzanne stopped dancing abruptly and sat down, the moment that our hands met in a clap, the moment our feet almost touched and Suzanne moved away, the moment Suzanne first caught sight of herself in the mirror, the moment she became aware of me reflecting her movement, the moment of the final handshake . . . these are all moments that occur in an instant. Too quick for words to catch, fleeting, transient, and ephemeral but laden with meaning and relation. The experience in psychosis is one of a body in pieces. A movement will happen and then it will pass and can never be repeated in just the same way but the experience is remembered, is retained in the part body/self which is slowly, over time, integrated into a whole body being.

SUMMARY

This chapter explores what dance movement therapy can contribute to the treatment of psychotic patients in psychiatric hospitals. It has emphasized that by working with the body, the dance movement therapist can address the heart of the problem in psychosis, that of the lack of cohesiveness in the bodily ego. The application of theory to practice is demonstrated through the presentation of a case. It describes the frustration and despair that was experienced by both the patient and the therapist when confronted with obstacles created by the very fact of working within an institutional setting.

REFERENCES

Balint, M. (1968) *The Basic Fault*, New York and London: Tavistock/Routledge, 1989.
Bernstein, R. F., O'Neill, R. M., Galley, D. J., Leone, D. R., and Castrianno, L. M. (1988) 'Body image aberration and orality', *Journal of Personality Disorders* 2(4): 315–22.
Bick, E. (1968) 'The experience of skin in early object relations', *International Journal of Psycho-Analysis* 49: 484–6.
Bion, W. R. (1957) 'Differentiation of the psychotic from the non-psychotic personalities', *International Journal of Psycho-Analysis* 38: 266–75.
Boss, M. (1979) *Existential Foundations of Medicine and Psychology*, London: Jason Aronson.
Bowlby, J. (1957) 'An ethological approach to research in child development' in J. Bowlby (1979) *The Making and Breaking of Affectional Bonds*, London: Tavistock.
Brazelton, T. B., Koslowski, B., and Main, M. (1974) 'The origins of reciprocity: the early infant–mother interaction', in M. Lewis and L. A. Rosenblum (eds) *The Effects of the Infant on its Caregiver*, New York: Wiley.
Cardone, S. S. and Olsen, R. E. (1969) 'Chlorpromazine and body image', *Archives of General Psychiatry* 20, May.
Casement, P. (1982) 'Some pressures on the analyst for physical contact during the reliving of an early trauma', in G. Kohon (ed.) (1986) *The British School of Psychoanalysis: The Independent Tradition*, London: Free Association Books.

Cox, M. (1978) *Structuring the Therapeutic Process: Compromise with Chaos*, revised edition 1988, London: Jessica Kingsley.

Davis, M. (1970) 'Movement characteristics of hospitalized psychiatric patients', in M. N. Costonis (ed.) (1978) *Therapy in Motion*, University of Illinois Press, pp. 89–110.

Dell, C. (1970) *A Primer for Movement Description: Using Effort/Shape and Supplementary Concepts*, New York: Dance Notation Bureau.

Dosamantes-Alperson, E. (1987) 'The function of kinaesthetic and kinetic imagery in the retrieval and assessment of internalized and transferential relationships of patients', in *Selected Presentations of the 22nd Annual Conference American Dance Therapy Association, Monograph No. 4.*

Fairbairn, W. R. D. (1941) 'A revised psychopathology of the psychoses and psychoneuroses', in W. R. D. Fairbairn (1952) *Psycho-Analytic Studies of the Personality*, London, Henley and Boston: Routledge & Kegan Paul.

Fisher, S. and Cleveland, S. (1965) 'Personality, body image boundary', in M. N. Costonis (ed.) (1978) *Therapy in Motion*, University of Illinois Press, pp. 162–78.

Freud, A. (1936) *The Ego and the Mechanisms of Defense*, revised edition 1966, New York: International Universities Press.

Freud, S. (1914) *Remembering, Repeating and Working-Through*, in *The Standard Edition of the Complete Psychological Works of Sigmund Freud*, Vol. 12, London: Hogarth Press.

——(1917) *Introductory Lectures on Psycho-Analysis*, Part 3. *S.E.* 16.

——(1923) 'The Ego and the Id', *S.E.* 19: 3–68.

Grand, S. (1982) 'The body and its boundaries: A psychoanalytic view of cognitive process disturbances in schizophrenia', *International Review of Psycho-Analysis* 9: 327.

Hinshelwood, R. D. (1987) *What Happens in Groups*, London: Free Association Books.

Kestenberg, J. (1975) *Children and Parents*, New York: Jason Aronson.

Klein, M. (1946) 'Notes on some schizoid mechanisms', in *Envy and Gratitude*, New York: Bell Publishing Company, 1975.

Lacan, J. (1977) *Ecrits*, London: Tavistock.

Lewis, M. and Rosenblum, L.A. (eds) (1974) *The Effects of the Infant on its Caregiver*, New York: Wiley.

Little, M. (1986) *Toward Basic Unity*, London: Free Association Books and Maresfield Library.

Mahler, M. S. (1968) *On Human Symbiosis and the Vicissitudes of Individuation*, New York: International Universities Press.

May, R. (1958) 'The origins and significance of the existential movement in psychology', in R. May, E. Angel, and H. Ellenberger (eds) *Existence*, New York: Basic Books, pp. 3–36.

Merleau-Ponty, M. (1962) *Phenomenology of Perception*, London: Routledge & Kegan Paul.

North, M. (1972) *Personality Assessment Through Movement*, London: MacDonald & Evans.

Pankow, G. (1961) 'Dynamic structurization in schizophrenia', in A. Burton (ed.) *Psychotherapy of the Psychoses*, New York: Basic Books, pp. 152–71.

——(1981) 'An analytic approach employing the concept of the "body image"', in M. Dangier and E. D. Wittkower (eds) *Divergent views in Psychiatry*, New York: Harper & Row.

Reich, W. (1945) *Character Analysis*, New York: Simon & Schuster, Turnstone Books.

Rosenfeld, H. (1971) 'Contributions to the psychopathology of psychotic states: the importance of projective identification in the ego structure and the object relations of the psychotic patient', in E. B. Spillius (ed.) (1988) *Melanie Klein Today*, Vol. 1, London and New York: Routledge, pp. 117–37.

——(1987) *Impasse and Interpretation*, London and New York: Routledge, 1988.

Sandler, J., Dare, C., and Holder, A. (1973) *The Patient and the Analyst*, London: Karnac Books, Maresfield Library, 1979.

Schilder, P. (1950) *The Image and Appearance of the Human Body*, New York: International Universities Press.

Searles, H. F. (1965) *Collected Papers on Schizophrenia and Related Subjects*, London: Karnac Books, Maresfield Library, 1966.

Segal, H. (1955) 'Notes on symbol formation', in E. B. Spillius (ed.) (1988) *Melanie Klein Today*, Vol. 1, London and New York: Routledge, pp. 160–77.

Siegel, E. V. (1984) *Dance Movement Therapy: Mirror of Ourselves*, New York: Human Sciences Press.

Spotnitz, H. (1985) *Modern Psychoanalysis of the Schizophrenic Patient*, second edition, New York: Human Sciences Press.

Tillich, P. (1944) 'Existential philosophy', *Journal of the History of Ideas*, 5(1): 44.

Winnicott, D. W. (1960) 'The theory of the parent–infant relationship', in (1979) *The Maturational Processes and the Facilitating Environment*, London: Hogarth Press and the Institute of Psycho-Analysis.

——(1962) 'Ego integration in child development', in (1979) *The Maturational Processes and the Facilitating Environment*, London: Hogarth Press and the Institute of Psycho-Analysis.

——(1971) *Playing and Reality*, Harmondsworth, Middx: Penguin, 1980.

Chapter 6

Imagery and metaphor in group dance movement therapy

A psychiatric out-patient setting

Kristina Stanton

INTRODUCTION

This chapter will discuss the use of dance movement therapy groups in a psychiatric setting. The main focus will be dance movement therapy groups which are run in community mental health centres, such as day hospitals and day centres which form part of out-patient treatment for adults. To provide a contrast to this, the chapter will make brief mention of how this approach would be modified for use with patients from hospital acute admissions wards.

Historical background

In order to appreciate the diversity of influences which form a dance movement therapy approach to working with groups of psychiatric patients, a glance backward to the development of group psychotherapy in psychiatry and to the early work of dance movement therapists is useful. Also of interest is the attention paid by psychiatrists, psychologists, and non-verbal communications researchers to the abnormal movement patterns which are characteristic of mental illness.

The use of therapy with psychiatric patients is a complex and controversial issue; some anti-psychiatry proponents, such as R. D. Laing (1971), believe that psychotherapy alone can alleviate the suffering of schizophrenics. Other schools maintain that treatment for such patients ought to be solely pharmacological, and that any type of psychotherapy may be positively harmful for people in serious mental distress. A contemporary understanding of mental illness, which views it as a phenomenon with a multifactorial aetiology (including both biochemistry and emotional conflict), enables us to take the forward-looking view that safe, supervised, non-intensive therapy is possible for such patients. The goals of such therapy are neither 'cure' nor any major restructuring of the personality. Rather, Yalom (1970) describes goals such as the improvement of patients' ability to form and maintain interpersonal relationships and the facilitation of their functioning as members of a group.

The last fifty years have seen a dramatic increase in the ability of psychotropic medication to control the symptoms which occur in serious mental illnesses, such as schizophrenia and major depression. Additionally, a small but significant number of psychiatrists and psychotherapists, as documented by Karon and Vandenbos (1981), have attempted to modify traditional psychoanalytic methods to treat individuals and groups of more disturbed patients using verbal therapy. Common themes in their work include the importance of repairing disturbed relationships, with parent figures as well as with siblings and peers. Also, they stress the need to attempt to understand the seemingly bizarre communication of such patients as symbolic; the garbled speech of the schizophrenic may make more sense if analysed in the same manner as a dream.

Interestingly, many authors stress the relevance of non-verbal aspects of the patient's behaviour which are assumed to illustrate the quality of psychological functioning from the patient's pre-verbal period of development. Non-verbal cues offer important insight into the underlying feeling state of the patient. The tradition of therapy for schizophrenic patients also stresses the need for the therapist to be aware of his or her own counter-transference, which in DMT is defined as the therapist's own emotional and bodily responses to the patient. Sandel (1980) stresses that access to the counter-transference may give valuable insight into what the patient is consciously and unconsciously feeling. Reflecting the patient's body movement, either with words or with the body of the therapist, is thought to 'clarify for the patient what he or she is actually experiencing' (Prouty cited in Karon and Vandenbos 1981: 31).

Dance movement therapy[1] in fact began as an attempt to use dance to make contact with severely regressed psychiatric patients, some of whom did not speak at all. Marian Chace (Chaiklin 1975), an early American pioneer of dance movement therapy, made some extraordinary forays into the world of the mentally ill when she worked at St Elizabeth's Hospital in Washington, where many returning war veterans were treated for what were described then as 'war neuroses' and would probably be described today as 'Post-Traumatic Stress Disorder'. She endeavoured to use her own body to reflect or mirror the patient's movement, so as to understand through her own experience what the patient's gestures might symbolize (Bernstein 1979). She developed a method whereby the group stands in a circle, each person taking a turn leading an improvised movement which the rest of the group follows or mirrors. This primary structure still forms the basis of much work done with psychiatric patients, and will be described below.

The complex task of interpreting movement is attempted on a number of levels, such as those described by Davis (1974). Movement a) may illustrate a patient's intrapsychic state or be an interpersonal communication to the therapist; b) will have a rhythm and organization which may evidence at which developmental phase the patient has encountered difficulty (Kestenberg 1975); and c) may have a metaphorical meaning; for example, a patient with sunken shoulders may later say that they feel they have the weight of the world on their back; another whose arms are held in a frozen position may feel that they are incapable of taking matters into their own hands.

Historically, the sometimes bizarre movements made by the mentally ill have attracted the attention of psychiatrists. With the advent of neuroleptic drug treatment, most of these abnormalities are no longer evident. Instead, movement disorders resulting from neuroleptics or anti-psychotic medication, such as akathisia (motor restlessness) and tardive dyskinesia (late-appearing disjointed movement), have come to characterize the gait of the long-term psychiatric patient. Recent research suggests that 'the distinctions between motor symptoms related to illness and those due to neuroleptics are blurred' (Nichols-Wilder 1987: 80). In the nineteenth century, it was fashionable for middle-class Victorians to view asylum patients from the galleries during what was known as a 'lunatics' ball': the strange posturing and extravagant gestures were something of a circus curiosity (Showalter 1985). Early psychiatrists, such as Bleuler, Kraepelin, Charcot, and Maudsley, attempted psychological and later neurological explanations for motor disorders such as 'catatonia' and the dramatic stages of hysterical attacks (Simon-Dhouailly 1986). In modern research, the difficulties of describing, classifying, and understanding movement pathology continue. Recent approaches stress that motor and thinking abnormalities in mental illness may have a common pathogenic basis (Manschreck et al. 1982).

Philosophical orientation

Dance movement therapy does not align itself with any particular psychological or psychoanalytical school; movement data can be invoked as evidence for a diverse range of psychological phenomena. Although in the UK Winnicott, Bion, and Klein, and the object relations tradition seem to be attracting a number of dance movement therapists (Holden 1990).

The present chapter seeks to apply object relations theory and existential and humanistic group psychotherapy approaches, with an important focus on the interpretative use of symbolism and metaphor in verbal and movement group process.

Theoretical foundation

Dance movement therapy in psychiatry appropriates ideas from two important sources: first, the psychological and psychotherapeutic treatment of patients, and, second, the interest in motor abnormalities of the mentally ill. Then it seeks to blend the psychological and the physical by understanding the non-verbal aspect of psychological health and attempting to utilize the expressive potential of movement in a creative form of psychological treatment.

TECHNIQUES

Goals

The goals of dance movement therapy with psychiatric out-patients resemble those of verbal group psychotherapy; the way these goals are achieved differs slightly, and there are movement level goals as well. The primary focus is to activate and motivate patients to use movement as a means with which to experience new ways of interacting with others. Furthermore, the movement yields imagery, and can so be interpreted as evidence of unconscious process in the group. Movement without words can also be analysed, and the communication contained within the quality of movement can be reflected back to the clients by the therapist. Improving a pathological movement profile cannot be considered an aesthetic task; rather, the dance movement therapist hopes that movement experience will extend the patient's expressive range of movement, in planes, shapes, and qualities. It is assumed that the non-verbal dimension illustrates intrapsychic pathology; therefore, making an impact on the movement level is assumed to affect overall psychological health.

With in-patients, the work is much more movement based and far less interpretative. Such groups aim at support, integration, and sealing over or dampening down the psychotic material which the patient produces. The use of concrete movement tasks for admissions ward patients can aid in facilitating clearer communication and non-stressful non-verbal interaction with other patients (Yalom 1983). Further, movement work can assist in improving short attention spans and re-integrating fragmentary or distorted bodily experience, such as the experience of the body being controlled by outside forces.

Practical aspects of the psychiatric setting

In order to function effectively, the dance movement therapist must have adequate therapy space, a supportive co-worker, and good relations with the staff of the community mental health centre in which he or she is employed. The room must be relatively spacious, and have curtains and doors which ensure privacy; nothing is less conducive to a therapy session than the threat of interruption or intrusion. The room should include enough chairs for everyone, and a large central space in which the group can stand in a circle and still move fairly freely. A group will generally include no less than five and no more than eight patients, plus a dance movement therapist and a co-worker (normally a psychiatric nurse, student nurse, or occupational therapist).

Since dance movement therapists currently mostly work on a sessional basis, it is essential that the co-worker be a member of the community mental health team who is familiar with the patients, and who has participated in the selection process for the group. Generally, when a dance movement therapist comes to work at a day hospital or treatment centre, they should provide an in-service presentation describing the DMT approach and indicating some criteria for client referral. Most therapists favour a mixed sex group of approximately similar ages and status; that is, at roughly the same stage in treatment, either in early assessment or in a period of lessening their dependence on the treatment centre. Patients for the DMT group can be drawn from most of the diagnostic groups which typically are seen in out-patient treatment, such as those assessed by the psychiatrist to be suffering from depression, schizophrenia (when stabilized on medication, and not floridly psychotic), personality disorders (e.g. borderline, narcissistic, etc.), or patients being treated for anxiety, phobias, anorexia, alcoholism, drug dependency, bereavement, or other psycho-social stressors.

Some day centres may demand that group membership be flexible or open to continual change, in which case the therapist and co-worker must be prepared to alter their goals and expectations to adjust to groups of this type (Yalom 1983). Ideally, the membership of the group is stable, though not closed; if membership drops below five, new persons are introduced. It is useful to do two open sessions for approximately ten patients, to familiarize them with the approach, and to get a sense of which patients may be unsuitable for a group; one can generally expect about a 30 per cent drop-out rate from these open membership assessment groups. In contrast, the acute admissions group may have the same membership for only a single session, making the primary focuses those of structuring interaction, extending movement range, and decreasing anxiety.

In out-patient work, a contract is made *with the remaining patients* for a DMT group of fixed period, usually between twelve and sixteen sessions. Here, it is important that other staff know who is in the group, and so understand that, even if patients are to be discharged, it is best if the patient continues until the end of the group. The fixed-term group allows the patients and the therapist to remain focused on the therapeutic tasks of adjustment, communication, and later separation. Short-term group therapy of this type is also economically sensible, and may allow lower-functioning members to master their anxiety about joining a group, because they know that it has a limited life span. It must be noted that out-patient therapy groups in other settings, such as those run in community centres or mental health drop-in centres (such as those run by MIND or similar voluntary organizations), may require a different approach, perhaps longer-running groups in which the aim is more to support clients in the community than to facilitate change in the level of interpersonal functioning.

After sessions four, eight, and sixteen (of a sixteen-week programme), it is appropriate for the dance movement therapist to report comments and insights about the patients to the key worker, or to the rest of the treatment team which may include psychiatric nurses, occupational therapists, social workers, psychologists, and psychiatrists. The therapist can give important information here based on non-verbal information gathered in the groups, such as observing that a depressed patient is appearing more grounded or more integrated, signalling a return to higher functioning, or that a person suffering anxiety is now able to gain more release in a particular movement warm-up. It is often helpful to attend meetings of all the staff concerned with a particular patient so that the team can assess which approach is most benefiting the client.

It is imperative for the dance movement therapist to have outside supervision from a qualified therapist, who may observe videotapes of the group, provided patients give their consent to be videotaped, or who may observe the group live. The importance of continual supervision cannot be stressed highly enough; without this, the therapist can become lost in a complex group process, or counter-transferential muddle, and knowingly or unknowingly inhibit the emotional development of the group. Additionally, work with more acute patients can be confusing and exhausting. Supervision is imperative for therapists attempting to work with this level of disturbance (Skove 1986).

Specific strategies

Since dance movement therapy is a type of therapy which relies heavily on improvised movement, it is important to attend to making the atmosphere of the group one of safety and security, which encourages the patients to experiment with new interpersonal behaviour and new ways of expressing themselves in movement. To this end, it is essential that the structure of the therapy group remain constant throughout the life of the group. Groups must meet at the same time on the same day, and begin and end on time. Depending on the level of the group, each session will last 1–1½ hours. Each group will include: an initial discussion, choosing some music, a structured warm-up led by the therapist, and then a process section, in which the main emotional work of the session takes place, followed by a group discussion which reflects upon the events of the session, and allows for closure of the session.

In the initial discussion section, each member in turn says how their week has been, and may list one good thing and one bad thing that has happened. For patients who tend to stick to concrete events, the therapist may ask, 'How have you been feeling in yourself?' to elicit a statement about the patient's emotional state of mind. After this, it is often useful to ask the patient to rate their week on a scale of one to ten, with ten being brilliant and one being awful. This allows the patient to reflect on this week in contrast with the last, and enables them to compare their state with that of the other members of the group. The therapist and co-worker also take a turn, though self-disclosure is kept to a minimum. The therapist must allow each person equal time and curb those who wish to talk at too great a length. In an admissions setting, the discussion will usually focus on introducing the patients to one another, and helping to relieve hospital-related anxiety and to orientate the patient to his or her new surroundings.

The therapist may summarize shared issues amongst the group, reflecting what several members may be saying about feeling stuck, or lacking motivation, or feeling frustration at the slowness of improvement in their condition. Alternatively, the therapist may reflect that, although the group's concerns are very diverse, everyone can appreciate none the less the situation of others. In this initial group discussion, the therapeutic factors are the same as those in verbal group psychotherapy. First, seeing other patients getting better instils hope in those who are struggling; second, being a useful member of the group is a corrective emotional experience and recapitulates the family grouping; third, after overcoming initial anxiety, members can develop socializing techniques which enable them to have more satisfying relationships inside and outside the group; and, fourth, expressing feelings in a group serves the purpose of catharsis or releasing emotional energy (Yalom 1970, 1983).

After this phase, the therapist encourages the group to choose some music, which can be from the therapist's selection or brought in by the group members. Interesting insights into the group process can be gained by observing how the group sets about making a democratic choice of music. The music, it must be stressed, is more for background than for dance. It is important to make clients feel comfortable in moving together, but the music should not be so rhythmic or overpowering that it determines the rhythm and quality of the movement in the process section. Popular music in groups with psychiatric patients may include current pop music, reggae, classical guitar music, African percussion, and many others. Choice of music should support rather than overwhelm free improvisation. Music which has little internal structure, such as experimental or New Age music, often encourages members to remain closed off, rather than facilitating interactive movement.

Once music is chosen, the therapist invites the group to stand in a circle, with the co-worker placed roughly opposite. The warm-up consists of a series of movements similar to those in a light exercise class or a beginners' contemporary dance class. A useful sequence to follow is: moving through the planes, vertical, horizontal, and sagittal (or diagonal), by stretching to the ceiling, touching the floor, reaching side to side, and forward and back. This facilitates exploration of the kinesphere. Depressed patients often have quite a limited sphere of movement, but this should not be verbally corrected by the therapist. Their range of movement improves in conjunction with their overall mental health.

In order to achieve the goal of expanding the clients' overall range of expressive movement, the therapist may invent characteristic movements which utilize the choreographic principles of Effort-Shape, developed by Rudolf von Laban (Laban 1948). These are the elements of weight, space, time, and flow. A sequence may incorporate, for example, for weight, walking and stamping; for space, reaching in various directions; for time, moving in slow motion and then with quickness; and finally, for flow, moving in a restrained way and then in a relaxed, easy way. Here, a professional training in dance movement therapy becomes essential to understand the movement of a patient. Range, restriction, expressive quality, interpersonal meaning, and symbolic meaning all need to be studied in detail, in order to understand movement and its use in therapy. For the acute patient, the warm-up may take up as much as half of the group; reorientating themselves to bodily experience can often be a great relief for the disorganized patient and help facilitate their participation in other ward-based activities.

In the main process section of the group, which may last up to half an hour, each member of the group (including the leader and co-worker) takes a turn initiating an improvised movement, which the rest of the group then follow or mirror. This can be an expansive, large movement, or a small gesture. The movements are not like those in mime, in which an action is presented, but similar to those in dance improvisation. The group should be encouraged to do anything, off the cuff, and not to prepare or plan their turn at taking the lead. The technique of shared leadership stresses the patient's growing autonomy, and allows them to gain a greater awareness of their own movement, by seeing it reflected by the group (Bernstein 1979).

At this stage the therapist encourages the group to free associate, both verbally and non-verbally, around each movement. The therapist may ask, 'What are we doing?', 'What does this remind you of?', 'How could we describe this with a picture?', or 'How does this one feel?' to elicit the group's verbal response. If one person started a movement in which they waved their arms gently, and then the group said this was like flying, or swimming, the therapist could get the group to clarify which of the two the movement most resembled.

In observing the other group members performing the movement, there is a pressure for the group to synchronize and for movements to become more standardized within the group. If the movement becomes most like flying, the therapist could ask the group to explore that quality, and ask, 'How are we flying?', to which a member might reply, 'through a storm' or 'over the mountain'. This might elicit further group imagery, and the therapist might engage the group in imagining, 'Where would we go if we were flying?', and the group members might say, 'I'd like to fly out of here', or 'I'm always flying into a rage', or 'I wish we could fly away to Spain'. The therapist consequently might interpret the group's behaviour as a sign that they want to become more independent and autonomous. Alternatively, the therapist might suggest that the group does not want feelings to 'take off' or 'land' on them without their being in more control. Imagery can thus be interpreted to a certain degree whilst the group is still moving, or explored in the final section of the group, when seated, during the closure discussion. There, the therapist might ask the group, 'I wonder what all that flying was about, or what sorts of feelings were inspiring that movement. Does anyone have any ideas?' It is important not to quash the unconscious process or interrupt the imagery and movement as it happens. However, it is important to assist the group in reflecting on their behaviour as it is happening, so as to prevent them merely releasing their feelings, rather than experiencing and thinking them through usefully. The therapist's task, therefore, is one of balancing between facilitation and interpretation, and observing the movement of the group carefully to gauge how involved it is in a particular movement or image. When involved, the group will evidence more Effort-Shape integration, and more complex group movement patterning which will alert the therapist to the fact that this particular theme is important to the group (Schmais 1981). In contrast, acute admissions patients will probably not be able to make use of the free association element; for them, this random material from the unconscious may emerge as a 'loosening of association', and is not helpful in enabling them to control their psychotic ideation. Sharing of the leadership should be retained, without the free association, as it still provides a structure for movement interaction.

Later the therapist may ask the group to extend a particular movement and explore it silently for a minute or two. This may yield a longer interaction and a more rich composite image from the group. For example, walking might become climbing which might become an adventure up a mountain, in which members will assign each other roles in the expedition, such as the guide, or an unexpected intruder. This more extended imagery will most fruitfully be analysed or processed by the group once it comes to a natural conclusion, or once the therapist has asked the group to use movement and words to complete the sequence. It must be noted that not all movements have imagery to accompany them; movement interaction without words, but connected to verbal process later in the group, can be equally effective in understanding and using the group process therapeutically.

With ten or fifteen minutes left, the group ends, perhaps using a movement given by the therapist to re-centre the patients and take them back into themselves, so that they are more composed and feel that the more expressive, imaginative part of the group has concluded. The group sits down again, on chairs or on the floor, to discuss the events of the day. Very often, themes which emerged in the introductory discussion will have expressed themselves in the movement; discussion of leaving, separation, or an imminent break in the group for a holiday period may re-emerge in the movement as an adventure or a perilous journey. In movement, the theme may manifest itself in a synchronization of members' movement, which signifies the group's attempt to cohere in the face of separation; conversely, they may fragment and use more individual style in a larger personal space during the process section. This might indicate a return to individuality, or possibly the disintegration of group cohesiveness.

After the group members have left the session, the therapist and co-worker discuss the session and make notes, keeping a record of observed movement patterns which particularly engaged the group, noting which members have changed their roles in the group and how individual and group movement evolved.

CASE ILLUSTRATION

The group which is described below ran for sixteen weeks, and was held as part of out-patient treatment in a day hospital (community mental health centre). It consisted of a dance movement therapist (the current author), a male student psychiatric nurse, Gary, as co-worker, and three male and two female out-patients. This was a relatively young group, with most members in their late twenties or early thirties. Three of the members (John, Eileen, Nigel) were diagnosed as schizophrenic, and were taking moderate dosages of antipsychotic medication; two lived in group homes, and one in a council flat. The other two patients, Paul and Elizabeth, were being treated for anxiety-related disorders. One of these patients lived at home and the other in a bedsit. These two patients also had individual counselling and used behavioural management techniques to deal with their anxiety. Two members did voluntary work in the community, in hopeful preparation for paid work, the rest were unemployed, largely as a result of their illnesses.

The session described here took place just after the Christmas break; the group had already been working together for about three months. The initial discussion centred on how everyone had coped with Christmas. The therapist said it sounded like most people coped with the holidays better than they had expected, but that there had also been some sadness associated with the time. She commented that people generally found holiday periods stressful as they were breaks from the usual routine. She added that her own Christmas had been all right, that her cat had kept climbing into the Christmas tree, and that everyone had overeaten. She rated her Christmas a six out of ten.

The group had difficulty deciding whether to have slow music, like Simon and Garfunkel, or fast music like the Beatles or Motown. Eileen said she wanted the classical guitar music so she could go to sleep. In the end, the group chose the Beatles, as they were a bit fast and a bit slow. The therapist commented that the group was in two minds about getting back to work; whether to ease into it or get off to a running start seemed an issue. The warm-up focused on all of the spatial planes and used Effort-Shape combinations. It accented being weighted and grounded, by using walking, stamping, and bouncy stepping. Eileen did not synchronize with the group, and Paul and Gary got into a joking competition about nearly stepping on each other's toes, which the group found funny.

Each person in turn led a movement. Gary dropped his head forward, and associated this with feeling ill when he had the 'flu. Everyone groaned, but doing his movement made them see how awful he must have felt. He said 'pass' to indicate that John, next to him, should take over the leadership. John started twisting from the waist, and then bent from the knee, so he was much lower. Everyone laughed, and the therapist wondered aloud what it might be like if we were all little people. Nigel said, 'like kiddies at Christmas!', and Eileen said, 'more like wallies'. John quickly moved up again, continuing his twisting side to side. The next person started something completely different; Eileen sat down on her bottom and started to spin around. The therapist asked what this felt like, and John said he felt dizzy, and Nigel said it was like being a helicopter. Eileen said it was only spinning, and abruptly stopped.

Nigel then took his turn; he stood up, brushed himself off, and said, 'Right, OK', and handed an imaginary package to the therapist on his left. She asked what it was, and he said, 'something delicate'. She handed it carefully over to Gary, who said 'aaahh!' as he took it. He whispered to John that it was explosive, and as John passed it to Paul he said, 'careful, it's semtex!'. We passed around the 'thing' until John decided that it was Gary's responsibility, and said he could keep hold of it. Here, the therapist noted that the patient was giving responsibility for containing the explosive feelings represented by the bomb to the student nurse. This was not interpreted directly, but put into the process. 'Why should he be the expert?' was the question posed. Nigel said that he might throw the bomb at the therapist, to see what would happen, and, whilst John smiled at this, the others looked uncomfortable at this thinly veiled expression of aggression. Paul, who ended up with the package, decided there was a bomb disposal unit in the corner and he walked over to the window and put down his imaginary package very carefully. He walked back, and the group looked at each other, wondering whose turn it was, and how that sequence had got started. The therapist said, 'Everyone seems relieved, does that mean it's gone for good?' The group was divided as to whether it was really defused or not. Conversation lagged, and the therapist realized it was her turn in the circle. She started a neutral walking movement, walking forward. The group soon synchronized in walking two steps forward and two back, all except Eileen, who did it the opposite way, and laughed.

John then took his turn; he sat down on the floor, and began to walk on his hands and feet, in the manner of a crab. The group was delighted with this novel way of walking, and they shimmied side by side, and pretended to kick into each other, or make surprised exclamations when they found someone was shuffling up behind them. The therapist asked, 'what are crabs like?' and Eileen quickly said, 'crabby, like you!'. Paul said crabs had hard shells, but were soft inside. This took the interest of the therapist, who wondered to herself what this image expressed about the group, and why they might choose this particular animal to symbolize themselves. John then said that they could all be on the beach, drinking beer by the bonfire. The group liked this image, and there were further comments made, and imitations of drunken crabs crawling along the beach. After a while, Eileen and Nigel said they were getting tired, and they sat down. Gary and John continued in a race for a while, and then, when the therapist, tired, sat down too, everyone stopped. The group sat on the floor, catching their breath. Paul said, 'that was a laugh', and Elizabeth said she thought the idea of herself as an old crab was only too right. This met with protests from Gary and John, who said, 'there you go again, moaning about yourself'. She smiled quietly.

The group got back on its feet, and the therapist commented that there were about twenty minutes left, and said they could start one more sequence of movement. Because the group was fairly co-operative that day, with people joining in on each other's imagery, and showing a high degree of synchrony in movement, the therapist could suggest more movement. If the group had been disorganized, the therapist might have introduced a prop, such as a lycra stretch cloth or a ball to focus the members' attention.

When the therapist asked for anyone with ideas, Nigel volunteered Paul, and, after some hesitation, he again offered a movement which resembled his earlier balancing on a tightrope. This time, he curved his arms more. The therapist exaggerated this curving, and the group also did larger movements. The process seemed stalled, as everyone stood on a spot, swinging their arms in a curve. The therapist asked if anyone could think of a way that we could all do this together; and after a moment, John moved his legs in tandem with his arms. Gary followed this, saying it was like 'walking funny'. This seemed to perturb John, but he continued none the less. The whole group started this walking, and walked out of the circle formation and around in a more complex pattern. The therapist asked, 'where might we be walking?', and Paul said, 'in long grass, or in a swamp'. Nigel corrected him, and said, 'No, we're lost in the jungle, and looking for each other'. Eileen queried, 'In a jungle? No, in a desert.' The therapist asked what we might find in the jungle, besides each other. John said, 'Snakes maybe!' and Elizabeth said 'I hope not!' Nigel crouched slightly, and said 'Lions!' The therapist crouched too, and then a few members of the group came closer into the circle, also crouching down. The therapist said, 'What can we do now?' and Paul said, 'Will the lion eat us?' He moved so he was behind Gary, the student nurse, and said, 'I'll stay behind you, so it eats you first!' Gary said, 'Thanks a lot mate' and the therapist said, 'Maybe we should ask Gary how he feels about being eaten first'. Nigel said, 'Maybe we should feed you to the lions!', whilst looking at the therapist. Paul objected to this, but Eileen smiled. Nigel said that the lion would probably eat both of us, referring to the therapist and the co-worker. During this time, Elizabeth had sat down on the floor, slightly away from the group.

The group continued to creep around, carefully, using great restraint, control, and focus compared with their usually disparate and heavy style of movement. There was a strong feeling of tension in the group. Nigel continued that only three in a hundred tigers were man eaters, to which the therapist added, 'or woman eaters'. 'Whatever', he concluded. The therapist asked again what the group was going to do about the threat of the lion. Paul suddenly said, 'run!', and he bolted over to where Elizabeth was sitting. She looked over at him. The rest of the group looked at the two of them, and the therapist asked, 'What will happen if we all run?', and John said, 'It will eat all of us then'. The therapist suggested that the group was saying that if they stuck together, they'd be better off than if they scattered. The group agreed. Nigel then said, 'Wait, maybe it's only a cub!' The group's tension and restrained body postures loosened perceptibly. Eileen said, 'Well that's good, then', and the group began to smile, and Gary leaned forward, saying, 'Here kitty, kitty'. The group then focused itself on stroking the cub. The therapist asked how such a cub could grow up to be a man-eater, and Nigel said that someone had tried to hunt it down, so it got angry. There was some discussion about what the lion would be eating if it didn't eat people; exotic grasses and smaller animals were suggested, before John said, 'That reminds, me, I'm hungry, what time is it?' Gary said it was ten minutes to twelve, and then the mood of the group shifted, back into being in the room, and out of the jungle. The therapist suggested that everyone come together again, and Paul and Elizabeth came back to the circle. The group concludeed with some easy stretching, and a centring exercise, in which widening and narrowing were used as a means of release. The group spent the last ten minutes discussing the session.

The therapist commented that they had been very active that day, and asked them to try to remember what movements and images had arisen. The group decided that the lion and the bomb were important. The therapist then asked if the group had any ideas on the meaning of these images, and if they showed how people were feeling. Paul said he was a bit worried about the explosive bit; the therapist asked why. He said he thought the bomb was a bit mean, and a bit dangerous. The therapist questioned whether there were any mean or dangerous feelings coming up, and what the group could do with them. She commented that it seemed that Gary had got dumped with the task of taking care of the group's dangerous feelings. Elizabeth said that everyone should deal with their own mean and angry stuff, but John said he reckoned everyone felt that way, sometimes. Nigel looked at the floor, and Eileen grinned and said she hated coming to the day hospital, and she would be glad when she didn't have to any more. This prompted John to say that it wasn't that bad, and it helped him to get his feelings out.

The therapist made some general comments about anger and frustration, and added that it was important that the group could share and acknowledge those feelings together, and that they would have to take responsibility for dealing with them, rather than expecting other people to do that for them. Elizabeth said she thought it was different watching people from doing things herself; she had got a bit annoyed about the lion and jungle part. She said that baby lions could still be dangerous, and that everyone forgot that. The therapist asked what the lion might say about the group, and John said, 'That we're starving', this made Eileen laugh, and the therapist enquired what sorts of things, besides food, the lion, or the group, might need, to which Eileen answered, food and shelter, and proceeded to tell us about her lack of curtains in her council flat. Paul said people needed money, and also other people sometimes. The therapist reflected that it was hard to go out and have to get all these things, simply to survive. The therapist said that the section of the group concerned with the crabs had seemed to her to show that the group did have things to share with each other which could be fun, not only angry or upsetting things. The group said they had felt good to get working again and doing something active after the holiday. Eileen said she didn't feel that good about getting back to things, Gary turned to her and rolled his eyes. The group finished, leaving to have coffee in the centre coffee bar before going home for lunch.

Commentary

After the group, the co-worker and the therapist discussed the group for about thirty minutes. They made detailed notes and reconstructed the early turn-taking movements, as well as checking observations with each other when comparing members' behaviour from this session and from the previous one. Finally, they spent time commenting on anything noticed in the session that the other might have missed.

There seemed to be a number of important themes which were becoming more apparent. Eileen's asynchrony with the group was more obvious; both in movement and in words, she set herself apart from the group (she had often used different levels, planes, and pace of movement, and once walked backwards and forward rather than vice versa, and commented that the group looked like 'wallies' at one point). We recognized that she was probably the least stable of the young schizophrenic clients, and that her recent move to a council flat had unsettled her. We noted that Elizabeth too seemed low, but attributed this to her not being able to identify with either Eileen or the female therapist, and to her feeling quite low over Christmas. We wondered too whether she was able to keep pace with the more physically demanding movements of the male members of the group. It was agreed that Gary, the co-worker, would actively mirror her lower level of activity in subsequent sessions, so as to draw her back into the group.

This particular group was readily able to use free association movement to develop symbolic themes. A number of emotional issues emerged from these themes, which might not have been raised had verbal group psychotherapy alone been used with this patient group. For example, 'explosive' feelings of frustration and anger could have been related to the holiday break; the group had been particularly cohesive about three weeks before the holiday. Furthermore, the way the group was dealing with those feelings was shifting; instead of seeing only the staff of the group as being able to hold or contain these feelings, the group was beginning to recognize that all of them shared such feelings. This realization aroused some anxiety in Paul. The group was concluding that they might help each other deal with these frightening feelings, first by feeling less isolated in their feeling, and second by exploring the source and aim of those same feelings. This theme of angry frustration re-emerged strongly later in the group process, when one member was refused a job, and felt enormously disappointed about this. At that stage, the other male members of the group could offer sympathetic support, which, whilst not taking away the cause of the feeling, did help that member feel less isolated in his struggle.

The symbol of the fierce lion who became a cub was interesting; it could be seen as representing the more dependent side of the group. The small animal in need of care and attention might resemble some of the unmet dependency needs of the group such as those described by Bion (1961). Assisting the group to see that they could help to feed each other, or just be able to ask for emotional support and to a certain degree obtain it from others, was a large step forward for these patients, who have great difficulties in forming satisfactory interpersonal relationships. Further, the symbolism of the crab, which has hardened defences on the outside, and is soft and perhaps vulnerable on the inside, seemed an appropriate image for the emotional lives of these group members.

The therapist also compared members' characteristic movements, to the movements of previous weeks. For example, Eileen's phrasing had become less clear, which was consistent with her being mentally less stable than before the holiday. John had used a quality of sharper timing to his movements; perhaps this was evidence of his attempts to be more clear and decisive about his own feelings, and about his family relationships. Nigel too had become more grounded in his movement than previously, shown in the way he used the element of weight in walking and stepping, and in his stamping his feet. The use of this element, which is correlated with a sense of self, probably illustrated his return to a less anxious state, now that the encounter with his relatives over the holidays had come to an end.

Finally, the therapist and co-worker noted their own counter-transference or emotional responses to specific patients. Here, Gary noted his lack of sympathy for Eileen, which he related to his feeling that her demands were too much for him (Skove 1986). The therapist noted Nigel's wishes to have her eaten by the lion and his threat to throw the explosive package at her, which caused her some anxiety about his aggressive feelings towards her. The therapist and co-worker discussed how some moments in the group had left them feeling disordered and disorganized; in one instance they were unable to recall whose turn it was to take the leadership! These sorts of feelings, present in verbal psychotherapy, may be exacerbated in dance movement therapy by the therapist's endeavours to share the patient's movement experience through mirroring (Skove 1986).

CONCLUSION

This group illustrates a number of important elements in a psychiatric out-patient group: the movement helps to motivate and focus the members, they learn to use the movement interactively and creatively, to explore new ways of being with each other. The symbols which emerge from the verbal free association give access to unconscious feelings, both within each member and for the group as a whole.

NOTE

1 This refers to how DMT began in the USA.

REFERENCES

Bernstein, P. (1979) *Eight Theoretical Approaches in Dance-Movement Therapy*, second edition, Dubuque: Kendall Hunt, 1982.
Bion, W. R. (1961) *Experiences in Groups and Other Papers*, seventh edition, London: Tavistock, 1987.
Chaiklin, H. (1975) *Marian Chace: Her Papers*, Columbia: American Dance Therapy Association.
Davis, M. (1974) 'Movement as patterns of process', *Main Currents in Modern Thought* 31(1): 18–22.

Holden, S. (1990) 'Moving together: the group finds a dance', *Group Analysis* 23(3): 265–76.

Karon, P. and Vandenbos, G. (1981) *Psychotherapy of Schizophrenia: The Treatment of Choice*, New York: Jason Aronson.

Kestenberg, J. (1975) *Children and Parents: Psychoanalytic Studies in Development*, New York: Jason Aronson.

Laban, R. von (1948) *Modern Educational Dance*, third edition revised by Lisa Ullman, London: Macdonald & Evans, 1975.

Laing, R. D. (1971) *The Politics of the Family and Other Essays*, London: Tavistock.

Manschreck, T., Maher, B., Rucklos, M., and Vereen, R. (1982) 'Disturbed voluntary motor activity in schizophrenic disorder' *Psychological Medicine* 12: 73–84.

Nichols-Wilder, V. (1987) 'Effects of antipsychotic medication on the movement pathologies of chronic schizophrenics', *American Journal of Dance Therapy* 10: 77–94.

Payne, H (1988) 'Dance movement therapy with troubled youth', in C. Schaeffer (ed.) *Innovative Interventions in Child and Adolescent Therapy*, London and New York: Wiley.

Sandel, S. (1980) 'Countertransference stress in the treatment of schizophrenic patients', *American Journal of Dance Therapy* 3: 20–32.

Schmais, C. (1981) 'Group development and group formation in dance therapy', *Arts in Psychotherapy* 8: 103–7.

Showalter, E. (1985) *The Female Malady: Women, Madness, and English Culture 1830–1980*, London: Virago Press.

Simon-Dhouailly, N. (1986) *La Leçon de Charcot: Voyage Dans Une Toile*, Paris: Imprimerie Tardy Quercy.

Skove, E. (1986) 'The psychophysical effects on the dance movement therapist working with a schizophrenic population', *American Journal of Dance Therapy* 9: 67–82.

Yalom, I. (1970) *The Theory and Practice of Group Psychotherapy*, third edition, New York: Basic Books, 1985.

——(1983) *Inpatient Group Psychotherapy*, New York: Basic Books.

Chapter 7

Alternatives in psychiatry
Dance movement therapy in the community

Monika Steiner

INTRODUCTION

This chapter discusses an example of care in the community for psychiatric patients. It reviews aspects of theoretical discourse on therapeutic communities from a social learning, existential, and psychodynamic point of view and relates these to DMT theory and practice. A case illustration of an ongoing twice-weekly DMT group with seven male adults in a psychiatric hostel, covering a period of ten months, will be presented. Its aim is to exemplify some of the practical issues and themes involved in setting up and leading a DMT group to give the reader an impression of one possible way to apply the insights and understanding of DMT to the field of mental health in the community.

The context

The subject matter of this material is a therapeutic community which has recently been established by a charity. Its original impetus stems from the present political climate in Great Britain which is based on a philosophy of change in mental health from 'custody to care' (Taylor and Taylor 1989), or, as it is better known, 'move into the community'.

With the closure of large psychiatric institutions the community is supposed to take over the humanitarian care of people labelled as mentally ill. Yet who is the community – family, social services, neighbours, strangers in the street? Many questions are raised by this policy. New concepts like management, efficiency, and decentralization have appeared. Resources are to be diverted away from the National Health Service to the statutory, voluntary, and private sector. These bodies will have to care for the old, the mentally handicapped, and the mentally ill. But are they able to do so or will this new policy be a way to cut the budget needed to care for the weak of society? Already there is increasing demand to come up with solutions and fill the gaps left by the planning of the national administration. I am convinced that the first to speak out against the inhuman aspects of institutions and the institutionalization of the mentally ill did not picture homeless schizophrenics roaming terrified in the streets of London.

The demand therefore for rehabilitation of people with psychiatric histories is on the increase. Sheltered halfway houses bridge the gap between psychiatric institutions and the community, thus facilitating a transition and helping to soften the impact of having to deal with the 'real world' after prolonged 'absence'.

Rehabilitation is the aim of the therapeutic community discussed in this chapter. It is designed to accommodate a maximum of eighteen residents. At present it has been running for ten months and gives shelter to nine residents. Each resident has a room of their own. Main meals are provided and eaten in a communal dining room.

The design of this therapeutic community is mainly based on a model of social work. This involves activating help for other members of the family, i.e. family meetings with social workers, parents' support groups, assuming that the reasons for the symptoms of the patient arise from the faulty family system. By taking away pressure from the resident it is possible to create the space necessary for them to increase their control over their own life. The staff is composed of residential social workers working on a rota basis to provide twenty-four-hour cover.

The official aims of the hostel are to develop and enhance each individual's ability to function independently, to help improve their communication and life skills. Expected length of stay in the hostel is between one and three years. The community's goal is to enable residents to move on, either to small group homes or to live independently.

Theories on therapeutic communities and their application to DMTT

DMT and therapeutic communities have one feature in common: a plentitude of different theories and approaches. These partly overlap, partly emphasize different aspects. None, however, is able to explain the phenomenon in toto. Three dominant schools of thought can be identified. Each is based on a philosophical frame of reference and accordingly underlines different aspects of the complexity of human existence: 1 the learning of behaviour within a social system, 2 the existential-holistic model, and 3 the psychodynamic approach.

1 The social learning approach

The social learning approach focuses on the patterns of behaviour the individual learns in coping with the environment. From this viewpoint, individual differences in behaviour result from variations in the conditions of learning that the person encounters in the course of growing up. This model stresses the importance of social and cognitive factors as well as the role of observation, i.e. vicarious learning, in determining behaviour (Bandura 1973). In practical terms this translates as 'A therapeutic community may provide a structured environment conducive to learning new, more adaptable, behaviours, achieving greater self-understanding and awareness and increasing self-responsibility' (Badaines and Ginzberg 1979: 74). It assumes that patients cannot perform social roles 'outside' in a satisfactory manner. 'Inside' they can try out new ones and be allowed to make mistakes without being ostracized. They have the possibility of behaving 'as if' and can therefore experiment with a wider range of options (Badaines and Ginzberg 1979).

In her book *The Management of Boundary Crossing* Angela Foster says:

One of the aims of therapeutic communities is to avoid through their social system the anti-therapeutic effects of institutionalization, the dehumanising and de-skilling which reduce a person's ability to cope with life outside the institution. The four main characteristics of this social system are: democratisation, permissiveness, communalism and reality confrontation. A fifth, implicit in the other four, is the large group, which is relevant for the management of the community as a whole.

(Foster 1979: 273)

One could say that persons who experience the negative effects of mental health institutions will have to de-programme themselves and adopt new sets of coping behaviour which will render them more able to deal with the demands of their lives.

In DMT, the group provides a system in which participants learn new ways of moving and behaving, just by observing the diversity amongst the members. They can also take up suggestions offered by the leader. These invitations range from focusing on breathing patterns to copying each other's gestures and postures as well as trying out completely new movement patterns. The participants therefore have the opportunity to learn either through their own experience or vicariously about new possibilities that may help them to cope better with their environment.

2 The existential-holistic approach

This endeavours to see the whole person with all their different facets. It aims to relate on all the different levels, from the practical/functional to the emotional and spiritual. In their chapter on 'Therapeutic communities and the new therapies', Badaines and Ginzberg (1979) discuss the implementation of creative therapies. They define the goal of therapeutic communities as follows:

> to facilitate realistic, open, honest communication and expression of feelings, as well as meaningful social interaction with greater satisfaction and security, to reduce anxiety and distortion of reality, increase the sense of worth and self-esteem, mobilise an individual's initiative, creativity and productivity.
>
> (Badaines and Ginzberg 1979: 74)

From the perspective of DMT this can mean: trying out a new movement, possibly the opposite of what has just been done, or the same movement, but bigger or smaller. If a safe climate is created within a DMT session participants can start to experiment. This is not as easy as some behaviourists may like to think. There may be a long history of emotional investment in the perfection of one particular style using a limited range of movements. When this is the case, and it often is with psychiatric populations, it is extremely difficult to change these patterns. To this end it is beneficial to encourage members of a group to imitate each other. Thus, by adopting other people's movements they learn to empathize with them and so expand their awareness of themselves in relation to others as well as extending their existing movement repertoire.

Encouraging group members to take responsibility for themselves demands an abdication of the traditional authority model, or at least some reduction of the hierarchical system. In a DMT session the circle is the basic figure. Everybody can move at the same time, unlike in a verbal group, where, ideally, only one person speaks at a time. When moving everyone is on stage. Thus one could say this form of therapy is democratic. On the other hand, the leader is extremely important. In a culture where people have forgotten how to move freely and spontaneously there exists a distinct danger that clients see the dance movement therapist as yet another person who is there to tell them what to do. This is particularly so for those alienated from their bodies, who have no strong sense of self and are seldom able to focus on their centre as a source of energy and inspiration.

The concept of empathy or 'being with' is central to establishing first contact and creating basic trust. It is usually the non-verbal rapprochement which determines the quality of the relationship between the therapist and the client. To 'be with' a very disturbed person can be demanding and challenging. It requires maximum awareness, opening one's antennae to receive often coded information without judging it or wanting to change it. Hobson (1979), describing his experience in a therapeutic community, expresses a philosophy which is strikingly similar to assumptions made for DMT:

The ideal state of a relationship is one of aloneness – togetherness. This is not static, but is continually recreated out of verbal and non-verbal conversations between people in a balance of stability and change with a rhythm of intimacy and distance. We need to be in touch, literally and metaphorically; but just as important, we need space.

(Hobson 1979: 238)

His metaphors touch on the heart of DMT. Touch and space, contact and rhythm, stillness and movement, these are the issues addressed in every movement therapeutic encounter.

3 The psychodynamic approach

This is based on the body of psychoanalytic knowledge with its emphasis on unconscious mental processes of individuals and groups. When applied, difficulties can arise from the tension between intellectual understanding of concepts and the understanding gained from personal experience of intra-psychic processes (Bettelheim 1983). This means that as long as issues like anxieties, resistances, and so forth have not been dealt with by the worker in personal therapy and supervision, their clarity is blurred and likely to be interfered with by their own unconscious defences. These barriers decrease the effectiveness of the helper and no amount of intellectual understanding can make up for a lack of personal insight. It is therefore important to work constantly on increasing awareness so as not to contribute to and collude with an atmosphere of denial.

A therapeutic community is a large group of people with a history of mental breakdown, in which communal living, with all its practical and emotional implications, is part of daily life. This group soon becomes the object of projections, which originate from the first group, the family. (This applies to residents as well as caretakers.) The underlying principle of a therapeutic community, as well as of any other group-therapeutic activity, is to trust in the healing, repairing powers of the group (Foulkes 1964).

Based on the assumption that residents suffer from a distorted perception of themselves and their environment, due to lack or distortion in their earliest experiences of 'being seen' by their caretakers (Kohut 1966), one can view the therapeutic community as a multi-mirror. Mirroring is also an important concept for DMT. The experience of being reflected on a movement level by a whole group of people can be powerful. It creates an opportunity to see oneself echoed by others, like being listened to and responded to by a living sounding board.

Movement and bodily contact are the currency of the earliest communication between infant and caretaker (Stern 1985) and they are the elements which are evoked in a DMT session (Holden 1990). The group becomes a substitute mother, where participants are able symbolically and literally to hold and nurture as well as be nurtured. This can only happen in an atmosphere of trust. Hobson (1979), however, cautions: 'In promoting a therapeutic living-learning situation, it is most important to distinguish between togetherness and pseudo-mutuality and between loneliness and aloneness' (Hobson 1979: 238), thereby reminding us to respect the privacy of human separateness.

A therapeutic community is an intense environment in which contradictions and difficulties easily arise. Boundaries need to be clear and not ambiguous. The boundary between the community and the outside world is an obvious one. The same rules do not apply in both of them. Care needs to be taken not to slip into a state of 'us' versus 'them', which promotes paranoia and can become a substitute for dealing with tensions and difficulties arising within (Bion 1961).

The therapist needs to define the therapeutic space of the DMT group carefully and be mindful to distinguish the group experience from the everyday one of the hostel. Existing contradictions are already difficult to tolerate and cause confusion. On the one hand, residents are given responsibilities with the demand to 'be normal', to cope with tasks set in a treatment plan, which aims to integrate the individual into normal society. On the other hand, in the DMT group, regressed movements and behaviours are tolerated and even 'played' with, i.e. exaggerated and explored. In a separate and contained space, held firmly and safely by the therapist-mother, rests the potential for individuals to feel accepted with all their madness. Then barriers can be lowered, reparation can occur, and change can take place (Winnicott 1971).

The body boundary (Schilder 1950) is in some ways the ultimate barrier between a person and the outside world (Laing 1976). Many residents still feel enmeshed emotionally with their families. To ascertain the 'real me' on a movement level helps to ground, stabilize, and encourage an awareness of a separate identity which many still struggle to achieve since their process of separation-individuation has been hampered by either impinging or neglecting parenting.

Winnicott (1971) realized that people searching for therapy have in some way an impaired ability to play. He also made the links between play and creativity which allow the juxtaposition of inner and outer reality. A 'new therapy' session, like DMT or dramatherapy, can work by temporarily removing the person from the world in which they live and creating a safer place (Badaines and Ginzberg 1979). This allows for fantasy and imagination to lead us in our play. Emotions can be expressed in ritualized ways, mock battles can be fought, intrusive 'mothers' pushed away, and longing transformed into a movement gesture. Stepping in and out of different worlds enriches and gives opportunities for exploration of difficult emotions.

Some borderline patients communicate through actions as well as words. Their bodies and movements become symbols for much of their feelings (Holden 1990). 'The difficulty in dealing with these patients lies not only in their difficulty in communicating with us, but also themselves' (Mute 1989).

According to Chaiklin:

The more disturbed an individual, the more dissynchronous and fragmented are their movement patterns. There is a lack of connection between mind and body, an irregular and sporadic flow of effort, a lack of gestural or postural change or unity, or gestures which are random, ritualized or distorted.

(Chaiklin 1982: 709)

She therefore suggests that the prime goal of working with psychotic patients is to aid body integration and awareness, strengthen a realistic sense of body image and either enlarge the vocabulary of movement or help control impulsive, random behaviour (Chaiklin 1982). Furthermore there is encouragement to explore the movements and use their energy, to become more aware of the underlying feelings to play with the symbols and enlarge a patient's choice in style and action.

With reference to communication, another important aspect of a DMT group session is the interaction between participants. 'Moving with' is a direct and immediate way of communicating on many levels at the same time. Object relations theories teach us the importance of the 'other' in our early development. In a group there are many 'others'. This intensifies individuals' emotional reactions to the group process. A group-analytic understanding helps to make sense of often bizarre ways in which participants relate to each other (Yalom 1983).

In summary, the relationship between the three approaches, with regard to DMT with the emotionally disturbed, can be delineated as a three-layered building. The basis is the existential approach. It provides the foundation. The experience of 'being with' is needed to create the relationship between the therapist and the client so as to establish the basic trust, which in psychiatric populations is often so undermined from earliest childhood. To achieve this is a demanding task. It requires tolerance of the anxiety which haunts the client and an awareness that this can activate the therapist's own anxieties. They need to be open to such anxieties within themselves in order to establish a non-verbal bond with the client.

The second layer is the social learning approach. It is particularly relevant for helping the very disturbed to ground themselves and be orientated in the reality that is accepted by the majority of their society. Working on this level the dance movement therapist needs to be directive, making suggestions in a non-threatening way, thus giving the tools which are needed for further explorations.

The psychodynamic approach is the last layer of the imaginary building. It assumes motivation and interest as well as a certain ego strength in the group participants. The search for their truth makes them look out for recurring patterns and, in spite of inner resistances, try to understand the unconscious forces which motivate them. The therapist needs to be centred and balanced within him/herself to listen to the many echoes that vibrate within, as a response to the multitude of conscious and unconscious expressions of the group. Then the therapist can voice the unspoken and so facilitate a process in which people can become more aware and therefore less at the mercy of their inner demons.

TECHNIQUES

The style of a session is as much determined by the leader's personal movement repertoire and preferences as by the other participants' movement range. Different participants like different movements. More important than anything else is to allow people the freedom to choose for themselves. In an environment of tolerance one can create the possibility of taking risks in the hope that these new experiences are 'good enough' and will carry over into everyday life. The participants therefore gain, either by immediate or by symbolic learning, more understanding about their predicament and new ways of coping with themselves in this world.

A dance movement therapist has to be extremely careful not to slip into the mode of instructor, which can be a tempting thing to do, in particular when faced with a group of depressed individuals who feel too hollow and empty to come up with any initiative. Also somehow people in our society expect to be taught how to move, since they are convinced that they themselves do not know how to do it. For the therapist to take on the role of a teacher would only increase patients' dependence on others rather than encourage self-expression. On the other hand, movement structures and sequences, when based on cues from the group, can be introduced by the therapist as a way of enlarging the existing repertoire, thus creating new possibilities of touching the emotional potential of an individual.

The principle of 'following the process', borrowed from psychodynamic group understanding translates into movement language as follows: the leader observes the movements of the participants and repeats certain movement patterns. This can be very small, everyday movement, like the tapping of a hand or foot. By suggesting to the whole group to follow it, the leader emphasizes and legitimizes each

participant, helping them to feel that they all have a valid contribution
to the flow of the group. This raises participants' awareness of each
other and facilitates a safe way to interact. The leader therefore treads
a fine line, finding the balance between leading and following closely
the existing process.

Therapeutic qualities of dance

People with severe emotional disturbances often have a sense of isolation
which words are not able to overcome. Moving their bodies is a concrete
starting point which helps to make contact first with themselves and
then with others.

A number of aspects in dance are central to the experience of DMT.
Moving with another person creates a feeling of togetherness which can
be difficult to achieve with words. This non-verbal communication,
called *synchrony* (Brown and Avstreih 1989), can be the first step in
building a bridge between two different worlds, the one of the client
and the one of the therapist. Group movement is even more powerful.
Since ancient times this medium has been used to help people cope
with difficult emotions, like grief or anger, to contain anxieties, to
give the individual a sense of belonging, and to create a channel of
communication which is so primal it touches on a person's deepest
sentiments (Spencer 1985).

The existing *energy* of a group will determine if people will do minimal
movements whilst slumping in their chairs, leap, stomp, or tiptoe
around the room, or gently sway from foot to foot, only slightly shifting
their body weight. The latter is a very simple action that everyone can
do, yet it is also a means of focusing upon one's centre, finding a
physical as well as an inner balance.

Music is an important medium which touches humans in ancient
parts of our psyche. Reactions to *rhythm* are almost involuntary and
contagious. One can find oneself tapping a foot to rhythmic music
without being aware of it. A steady beat can help to provide a safe
environment within a group to express repressed and taboo emotions.
This often happens in a stylized manner. An emotional outlet or catharsis
of feelings used to be, and in certain ethnic groups still is, part of the
mental hygiene which prevents the bottling up of unwanted emotions.
Rhythmic movement also facilitates a strengthening of a sense of
self by emphasizing our contact with the ground and re-affirming
our connectedness within ourselves and with this world through
gravity.

Rituals help to alleviate anxiety. They provide a framework, in which
a frightened person holds on to the familiar in order to contain difficult
thoughts and feelings. They are also useful in clarifying the beginning

and end of a session, therefore helping with transitions, and signify a boundary between being in or out of therapy.

It is possible with movement to assert *body boundaries*, often distorted in psychotic and borderline patients. Basic assumptions like where do I start and where do I end, experiences the baby has to deal with when it learns how to differentiate itself from the rest of the world, are taken for granted by most people, but underdeveloped or damaged in the psychotic or borderline person. Simple movements like stroking or patting their bodies help to strengthen their perception of their bodies and therefore of themselves as individuals.

Touch of self and others is loaded with associations, from care and nurturing to violence, abuse, and sex (Willis 1987). It therefore has to be used with mindfulness and caution. If encouraged at the right moment it creates the quality of nurturing which so many have never experienced or, if they did, did not get enough of. There exists the danger of creating a self-perpetuating pattern which in the end is not therapeutic but becomes an end in itself, not bringing the client any further along the therapeutic journey. On the other hand, it also elicits powerful sensations which can be healing.

A dance movement therapy session

If I were to compare a DMT group in the psychiatric hostel I work in to some type of music, I would think of a jazz session. The beginning and ending are fixed, all the rest is improvisation. Everyone gets a chance for a solo whilst being supported by the rest of the band. When the players jar, dissonances are created; at other times harmonies prevail.

A DMT session starts with a warm-up to help participants make contact with body parts and get more in touch with themselves. For the leader this initial part helps to gauge the atmosphere of the group and the moods and states of the different individuals.

Different levels of energy bring forth different movement patterns amongst group members. By finding ways of 'moving as the other does' we come closer to the emotional experience involved in the carrying out of a particular movement or posture. This then elicits verbal and non-verbal reactions and the 'improvisation' may start. Themes develop that focus on one particular participant, their mood and movements, or a quality of the interaction between two or more participants. These can take the form of images that arise from the pooled group unconscious, triggered off by the common group activity. Ideally the group recognizes and acknowledges these, to understand and to become more aware of these unconscious forces. In reality a lot of things can happen at the same time and are too fast or elusive to be dealt with fully. Another possibility is that the group is so depressed and fragmented that we do not get beyond the warm-up in the first place.

Besides the abreaction or catharsis of feelings and the working on and through emotional themes, I want to mention one more factor which is often forgotten. Zorba the Greek danced when he was sad, but he also danced out of joy. Dancing, moving one's whole body, is essentially a pleasurable experience. It is this knowledge which we can share with our clients. Moving together as a group suggests a new-old way of making contact with one's physical, mental, and spiritual self and so confirming one's feelings of being alive.

Towards the end of a session we often have relaxation, in which everyone is on their own with their body, mind, and soul. Afterwards we sit in a circle on the floor and share how participants feel or any other thing they want to mention. This is like a period of transition, from a non-verbal to a verbal, from an instinctive to a cerebral mode of being, where movements and emotions are contemplated and translated into words, experiences clarified, and understanding deepened.

Finally we all get up, hold hands, and formally bring the session to an end. Then each participant closes their hands in front of their chest and with a little bow everybody thanks everybody else. It is often those last moments, when in some ways it seems to me that we have achieved a sense of honesty and togetherness, which are so precious and hard to describe in words.

CASE ILLUSTRATION

The greater part of the material now presented is what I learned from direct contact with the residents of an all-male therapeutic community in twice weekly, one-and-a-half hour DMT sessions. In the following word pictures the focus will be on physical impression, relevant background information, outstanding qualities, and the interaction in the seven-member group.

Nigel

Nigel, at 47, is the oldest resident in the hostel. He is tall, with greying hair, recently dyed to black. A slightly protruding lower lip combined with a nasal twang and deep furrows on his forehead produces an impression of doom and gloom. Only the twinkle in his eyes gives away his sense of humour. His sunken chest seems to rest on long legs without too much of a transition. He dresses formally in jackets and, often stained, trousers.

Nigel was diagnosed as schizophrenic at the age of 38, has had eight hospitalizations and stayed in different hostels for the last six years. His ageing mother lives under impoverished conditions in a council flat. She was lobotomized for depression when Nigel was at primary school. Nigel is divorced. Presently he attends a day centre five days a week doing industrial therapy. That means putting cutlery into boxes.

One of his symptoms is begging for a cigarette or ten pence. At times of stress he has episodes of conversations with God and out of the body experiences.

Nigel usually starts a DMT session by complaining about his mental or physical condition, like tension in his forehead or a bad back which will prevent him from participating fully. Then he slumps in his chair with closed eyes. In the course of one session he usually drifts out of the room several times. Mostly he comes back, sometimes he does not.

In spite of his, at best, sporadic participation in the group's movements, he can suddenly jump into the middle of our circle and show us complicated dance steps like the Samba or a Russian folk dance. Moving together with the rest of the group he relates little to other residents of whom he can be quite inconsiderate. After joining in for a short while he will stop to sit down, turn away, or leave the room. He is institutionalized, needy, and emotionally young. This expresses itself in his longing for touch. Like an infant he wants attention and contact. He may not participate actively for a whole session, yet when we close, i.e. hold hands in a circle, he will join in.

Patrick

Patrick is 30 years old, but looks like 13. He is small and thin, his whole body taut. His complexion is fair; blue watery eyes manage to stare with great intensity at nothing in particular. His face is like a mask, skin tightly streched over bones, expression frozen. When he smiles, which happens rarely, his whole face lights up. He dresses tidily and his straight back and politeness remind one of a perfect little gentleman. The only flaw in his appearance is his socks: most of them have gaping holes.

At the age of eleven he was traumatized by his father's sudden fatal heart attack. Shortly afterwards he again witnessed death when he saw his grandmother die. Then Patrick was sent to boarding school, since his mother, who herself had a history of psychiatric hospitalizations, could not cope. After failing his final exams at university, he had his first breakdown and since then has lived in different therapeutic communities, but was never hospitalized.

When asked about his well-being he mostly snaps back: 'Thank you, I am very relaxed.' At times his eyes well up, yet he laughs at the same time. Sometimes he freezes entirely and gazes into space. Then he exudes a sense of panic and of 'being on the edge'.

His movements are stiff like those of a wooden doll, on two planes only, like arm swings from side to side or forwards and backwards, his breathing is shallow. He seems weightless, without any sense of gravity in his body, and cannot feel his centre which is so important to one's experience of identity. One can only speculate about how empty he feels.

The most striking feature of his behaviour in the DMT sessions, which he attends regularily, is that he copies my movements with an amazing degree of accuracy. It seems as if his limbs are linked with invisible strings to my body. It may be that this movement relationship has become like an autistic shape (Tustin 1986) which gives Patrick a safe enough structure to make his participation in DMT possible. Any exercise with too many changes or possibility of improvisation seems to puzzle and confuse him. He talks little as if all his efforts are directed towards holding himself together.

Jeremy

He is 23 years of age, medium height, with round lifted shoulders and a hunched back. Thinning brown hair is meticulously attended to. A face with shining eyes, sensuous lips, and peeling skin completes the picture. He suffers from allergy and eczema. Underweight, he seems child-like and feminine. Small feet, loosely attached to frail ankles, appear to have ethereal contact with the ground at the best of times. His hairy chest, however, is the source of some contemplation for him. (He draws himself as a big ape!) Jeremy's intelligence is above average. He does not take any medication.

Jeremy gets into a push–pull pattern with his domineering mother, which until recently has rendered him unable to leave home success-fully. He has been hospitalized once for depression.

His anxiety leaks through in talking obsessively, pacing, and checking of doors and windows. He 'gets stuck' in his room and, more often, on the loo.

Jeremy has little movement range and imagination. When sitting he coyly crosses one leg over the other and swings the raised foot backwards and forwards. Standing up, he continues the same move-ment with his whole leg or swings his arms. His torso is stiff and uninvolved.

Jeremy's insights in the group process contribute valuable images and associations. In some sense he is the mouthpiece of the group. Verbally he can address other participants directly. Non-verbally he is wary of touch. A split can be perceived also in the love–hate relationship with his mother which he transferred onto the group and me, as its leader: DMT is either fantastic or useless. His patterns of participation in

DMT change in accordance with the frequency of his visits to his mother.

David

He is 30 years old, of medium height, stocky features, with a little pot belly. Round blue eyes can smile at you winningly or glare at you sulkily. He manages to combine rounded shoulders with a seemingly spineless lower back.

He has one younger sister, an intrusive father, and an absent mother. With two prior hospitalizations he has had experience of most medical treatments available. Convinced that the source of his problems is neurological, he takes medication against depression. He was diagnosed as suffering from an obsessive-compulsive disorder.

David has difficulties getting up in the morning and 'gets stuck' in his room with obsessive rituals: he has to bang his head against a wall and pick up things from the ground. (This prevents him from going out on his own.) At times he touches his penis, as if to check it is still there.

He seems like a 3-year-old, ready to throw a tantrum and not surprisingly in DMT he likes jumping and stomping his feet. When he is in a good mood he can move on more than two planes. Then he almost dances and is able to initiate but, usually after some time, he will stop himself. A distorted relationship to his body transpired in the course of time. Moving makes him more aware of his sensuality/sexuality. He feels so threatened by these sensations that he gets anxious and has 'bad thoughts' of an aggressive and sexual nature, mostly directed against female staff. Then he has to leave the room. Quite often though he manages to come back. He talks about his ambivalence towards the movement group and his fear to 'give all of himself'.

Billy

Billy is 22 years old. The youngest and most recent arrival to the hostel. Tall and thin, he looks like a twisted corkscrew: all knees, fingers, and elbows. His co-ordination is impaired for motoric/neurological reasons. A small head sits on a long neck twisted slightly to the left, like a young bird. He looks shyly out from behind thick, usually dirty glasses. The hair is cut short with small bald patches, which he inflicted upon himself in a self-destructive rage. His shirts are buttoned up tightly, slightly strangling his neck, the sweaters elongated, because Billy pulls them down between his legs. Originally diagnosed as having 'learning difficulties' he has not entirely mastered the art of writing clearly, but he can read and is intelligent.

A sadistic father has abused him from an early age scarring him physically and emotionally.

Billy cannot touch his belly, fingertips pointing towards his chest instead of feeling his abdomen. He is afraid of AIDS. He is afraid of touch, afraid of the group, and afraid of life. His movements fluctuate between a very young, almost baby-like manner to utter frustration and aggression, which can lead to violent outbursts. He likes stomping his feet and makes fists to beat himself with. He seems delighted when I suggest others follow his movements. When anxious, an unfiltered stream of words gives the impression of a traumatized and frightened individual desperately trying to cope. At other times he shows a high degree of perception and insight into his own and others' behaviour.

In the group he behaves like a victim, expecting to be bullied and kicked. When we form a circle, Billy turns slightly sideways and looks away from the middle, and when we hold hands he can start talking about hot countries, the danger of being stung by mosquitoes and catching malaria.

Victor

Victor is 31 years old, of medium height, has red hair, bright skin with lots of moles, and sweats profusely. He chain-smokes, has a constant chest cough and yellow tobacco-stained fingers. He dresses formally, his trousers pulled up high, giving a glimpse of his underpants which are pulled up even higher.

He arranges his dental appointments at exactly the same time as the DMT group. The few times he has participated he showed regressed behaviour, like constant rocking. He joined group movements only sporadically and often just lay down shutting his eyes. All the signs were saying that he finds this group difficult.

Roger

Roger is 33 years old, tall and thin. His posture seems like a question mark.

His most outstanding feature is that he hardly talks, but beckons with one finger if he wants something. In spite, or because of, this silence he can have a powerful effect on others. After seven months of ignoring my invitations to DMT groups, he has started to participate in the relaxation part of the session, after which he silently folds his mat and leaves the room.

The other two residents, Paul, 29 years of age, and Desmond, 23 years old, do not participate in DMT as yet.

The process

In the early stages of setting up this DMT group I had to introduce the concept of DMT to both staff and residents and I was viewed with slight suspicion, curiosity, and amusement, if not outright hostility. This ambivalence expressed itself mainly in the frequency of participation of residents and the amount of help I received from staff to coax residents to participate in the group.

At that time I invested the greater part of my energy and creativity in inviting people to the sessions and, once they were inside the room, trying to keep them there. Nigel in particular drifted in and out constantly. I sometimes wondered if some people were not too institutionalized to have any kind of therapy at all. It was clearly an effort just to be in a room together. At times this achieved absurd proportions: for example, once I started a session with one member of staff and four residents. Slowly one resident after another drifted out of the room until I was left with my co-worker and a circle of empty chairs contemplating the usefulness of ourr existence. For ten minutes we were 'safeguarding' the therapeutic space. Gradually one after another returned and we were able to move together again.

What I sensed in our initial sessions was despair and fragmentation. Often, before setting out for the hostel, as Levy (1988) describes, I felt depressed and burdened by the knowledge that if I did not go in and run this group it would not happen at all.

The movement range of the residents was limited. What seems a little task, like lifting arms or swinging them from side to side, appeared complicated and demanding. There was little, if any, interaction between participants. The greater part of the sessions was spent on the warm-up, making contact with body parts.

There was minimal initiative, Nigel and David were the most inventive. Both repeatedly suggested some movement for others to follow, but when we all did it, they would stop moving, leaving the rest of the group at a loose end. David initially had difficulty participating at all, because he had 'to pick up things' or rearrange them. Once, the whole group was encouraged to touch objects in the room and explore them, thus turning his obsession into a group activity. In some ways it was easier for the group to connect to objects than to people. Patrick, for instance, rarely made eye contact with anyone, Nigel in particular and other residents in general related to me only, rarely to each other, and sometimes there seemed to be a competition for my attention.

While we were waiting for everyone to gather I would start a session by asking people how they felt in their body. Nigel often described feelings of disintegration, others talked about their body as if it were not their own, reflecting their feelings of being alienated and out of control. One of my frustrations was about people's inability to follow movements I thought would be beneficial to them. This taught me the need to listen better, observe more closely, and more patiently improve my ways of empathizing, therefore challenging myself rather than others. (Verbally I encouraged any movement people made.)

For a long time the group seemed dependent and regressed. Slowly, disturbed patterns rose to the surface. These, after a long period of acceptance, could be verbalized and start to enter into an individual's consciousness.

When Patrick 'froze' and would not respond to any invitation from myself or others, the group needed to contain his anxiety as well as the anxiety it triggered off in the rest of us. Sometimes he 'defrosted' all on his own, sometimes a gentle repeated invitation to participate helped to bring him back, so that towards the end of a session he 'melted' and joined in the relaxation and closure. It took months of building up a relationship and the trust necessary to enable me to ask him what happens for him when he freezes. From his answer I understood that he feels extremely self-conscious, but I think this is not the whole story. It transpired that he had 'heard' me calling him all sorts of names. Interestingly enough another resident challenged him by asking if it was possible that he had imagined those voices.

A typical scenario of the group in its early days would be Nigel complaining of tiredness, slumping in his chair, David curled up on the floor with his back to the group banging his head on the ground, and Jeremy talking incessantly, fiddling with window locks and door handles, insisting that he could only move to 'his' music. Faced with this reality I wondered sometimes if I was the right person for the job.

Music evokes emotions, memories, and associations. It contributes significantly to the holding framework of the group activity. Other aspects of holding are my verbal interventions. These are suggestions to try out new movements. More interpretative statements acknowledge the mood of the group or that of an individual.

To my surprise I felt for a long time that it did not matter so much what I said but how I said it. I had the sensation that my voice was holding, soothing, and comforting, especially so in relaxation.

I always asked people for their associations to our movements. Sometimes they came up with an image, sometimes not, sometimes they all talked at the same time. Images that emerge from the pool of the group unconscious are often powerful symbols for emotions and provide material to play with and eventually help translate movements into words and thus facilitate the process of unfolding increasing awareness.

One image, appropriate for the early stages of this group, which cropped up time and again, was of a baby. Others were a wobbly man and puppets manipulated from outside. The feelings expressed were caution, ambivalence, disjointedness, and fragmentation. The atmosphere was often heavy and quite desperate. My task was to provide the holding environment for trust to develop and to contain the anxiety which accompanied the great change of moving into this new and challenging community. Once, at the beginning of a session, one resident remarked: 'We look like a family that has moved into a new home, but does not have the right furniture yet.' This image combined the feelings of alienation with the seeds of group cohesiveness. Thus the DMT group reflected the goings on of the hostel like a microcosm.

Incidents which strongly affected the group were staff-turnover, a recurring phenomenon, and holidays of workers. At these times residents verbally and non-verbally expressed their fears of getting attached, feeling abandoned, powerless, and manipulated. Their upset revealed itself in the to-ing and fro-ing in and out of the room, disjointedness, disturbed, regressed behaviour, and talk about desertion, death, and despair. My own holiday brought forth the image of being in a tomb gliding off a ship into the sea. On my return hope was symbolized by mats turning into magic carpets. Only Patrick made angry movements.

In following sessions the struggle of trying to contain people in the room for the whole session continued. I started to leave more space for verbal sharing at the end of the session after the relaxation. The latter, being the least demanding part of the session, became the cue to call back people who had left and not yet returned. They could then participate and stay throughout the verbal sharing and closure. So even when the atmosphere throughout the movement part of the session was disjointed we could gather again as one group. Thus a moment of stillness was followed by a moment of togetherness.

Shortly before the official house-warming party the group, for the first time, danced together joyfully and in synchrony. The image of a boat arose. The next session participants talked about feeling guilty after too much pleasure. They felt very old again and could only stretch, yawn, and curl up. The moment of togetherness came when residents started to sing old children's songs. Only months later could they verbalize the feelings already expressed non-verbally long before: 'we may be old in body, but we are really very young in mind.'

It seemed like a sign of growing trust when participants started to express more of the anger stored within. They found ways of venting their frustration in punch-like, clapping, and stomping movements and sometimes even shouting. An evocative image that emerged was Mike Tyson the boxer. When Jeremy complained of obsessive thoughts, which prevented him from stopping talking, I asked him to translate them into movements. His response was a crescendo of fists, shaking violently, and kicking movements. So he found ways of physical outlet for his nervous mental energy and was eventually able to contact some of the depression which was underneath his anger. Then he could even allow the group to hold him in the middle of the circle and rock him soothingly.

David and Billy had outbursts of frustration and anger, throwing tables or chairs in the hostel. Echoes of these incidents were reflected in the DMT group interaction: residents non-verbally refused to form a circle by either turning away, sitting down abruptly, or leaving the room. Later on they became more courageous at expressing their anger with each other and we could play at accidentally 'bumping' into each other.

After about five months I wrote in my notes: 'The group seems to move on in its development.' This was following the residents' spell of giggling during relaxation, which created the atmosphere of a boys' school dormitory rebelling against teacher. An image that came up during that time was a battleground between residents and authority, i.e. staff. Another possible interpretation was their struggle with inner authority, which seemed to relax its grip just a little.

Over time the group found more courage to experiment with movements like rolling on the floor. Crawling on all fours brought about lots of laughter and associations. From being cats we turned into dogs. This caused Nigel to lift a leg, grin and ask: 'What am I doing now?' Talking about bodily functions as if they are something normal was clearly a shock for some of the participants, especially the phobic ones who lock themselves in the loo with endless rituals. The humour and hilarious laughter of the other participants worked like a saving grace and gave more human proportions to 'this very serious matter'. Playing at being animals allowed Billy to become a baby monkey. He immediately hid underneath a table and even though he was smiling, clearly behaved like a frightened little animal.

As would be expected in a group of young males sex was an issue foremost on their minds. The majority had no sexual experiences with a partner and for most of them the whole subject was loaded with a mixture of natural desires, irrational fears, and fantasies. The images produced were the Exorcist and Dracula symbolizing the monstrous feelings lurking in the unconscious.

Increasingly residents started to verbalize their feelings of confusion, longing, shame, and fear. They would share their desire to find a partner and wonder if they would ever do so. David talked about his fear of exposing himself, Billy how he had attacked himself, piercing his penis with a dart, Nigel mentioned his ex-wife.

Lastly I want to share the memory of one session which, like so many others before, started with low energy and people expressing tiredness and exhaustion in words and movements. For what seemed a long time we stayed with small repetitive movements, patting the body, clapping hands. Then I introduced my circular band, made of old ties strung together. Everyone held it in one hand and we made some round movements with it. Asked what we were doing, Nigel said 'stirring' and Jeremy added 'in a cauldron'. Encouraged to add ingredients Nigel put in his sorrow, Jeremy his mother, then me because I had annoyed him by changing 'his' music, David added his confrontation, and Billy his anxiety. Thus the group had created a container for the difficult feelings each person experienced.

CONCLUSIONS

The DMT sessions I have described in this chapter are essentially the story of a group within a group. This means that the milieu is very important. It provides another, second container, like a concentric circle, around the DMT group. The therapist, as a member of a multi-disciplinary team, is part of a continuously changing web of relationships between staff and residents. One possible pitfall is the lack of appropriate communication due to personal insecurities, ambivalence, and the different background and philosophies between the professionals involved. Thus, instead of sharing complementary knowledge and skills, it is easy in contributing to the environment to add to a sense of fragmentation and conflict the residents already experience within themselves. A sense of trust and support within the team needs to be achieved, a common language found, to make it possible to provide the environment which gives a real alternative to the solid identity of the asylum with its clear boundaries (Taylor and Taylor 1989).

It was my policy to encourage staff members to participate in the DMT sessions. This was helpful in two respects. A positive relationship could develop between myself and the participating member of staff. Secondly, it contributed to the generation of a trusting holding environment in the group as a whole and so helped to deal with some of the problems that were bound to arise in such an intense environment.

First and foremost was the need to contain the anxiety generated by people who are afraid of mental breakdown. Because this fear is founded in reality (most residents having had psychiatric histories), this is a formidable task. Psychotic or borderline people have powerful ways of projecting their feelings onto others, sometimes in physical ways, and they often activate our own primitive feelings. This is particularly so in DMT since by its own definition the starting point is non-verbal communication. Thus a primary task in establishing this DMT group was to recognize how this atmosphere of fear affected me and, secondly, to keep analysing the counter-transference so that I could create the necessary therapeutic distance. Only in this way could I stay open to non-verbal messages and use them as signals which helped me understand and empathize with the residents and so establish a therapeutic relationship with each individual. Movement was the vehicle which created the structure in the sessions: it aided the process of grounding and centring and opened possibilities for symbolic expression, communication, and interaction.

One example of counter-transference was my need to idealize the residents, endow them with more potential than they possibly had. In retrospect I can see that this was a defence, my need to feel omnipotent and so fight off the feelings of incompetence and helplessness in the face of a frustrating reality. It was difficult for me to accept that, for whatever reasons, residents were severely handicapped and trapped in their self-defeating patterns. From a diagnostic point of view it is interesting to note that those residents who rarely participated in the DMT group were the most vulnerable and had relapses with spells of hospitalization.

I had to learn to accept residents' resistance and ambivalence and to adjust my expectations of what was realistic to hope for a client group as fragmented as this one. Residents were at various stages on the continuum between sanity, coping, and breakdown. Mutual support was nevertheless building up slowly.

Therapeutic communities like day centres, can provide a bridge between the psychiatric hospital and more integration within the community. Inter-relatedness between models which have different starting points can, like a building, together provide one theoretical frame of reference for DMT to offer an alternative to conventional psychiatric care.

REFERENCES

Badaines, J. and Ginzberg, M. (1979) 'Therapeutic communities and the new therapies', in R. D. Hinshelwood and N. Manning (eds) *Therapeutic Communities*, London: Routledge & Kegan Paul.

Bandura, A. L. (1973) *Aggression: A Social Learning Analysis*, Engelwood Cliffs, NJ: Prentice-Hall.

Bettelheim, B. (1983) *Freud and Man's Soul*, London: Chatto.

Bion, W. R. (1961) *Experiences in Groups and Other Papers*, London: Tavistock.

Brown, J. and Avstreih, Z. A. (1989) 'On synchrony', *The Arts in Psychotherapy* 16: 157–62.

Chaiklin, S. (1982) 'Dance therapy', in *Anthology – Basic Collection*, ed. staff team, Department of Education, University of Haifa.

Foster, A. (1979) 'The management of boundary crossing', in R. D. Hinshelwood and N. Manning (eds) *Therapeutic Communities*, London: Routledge & Kegan Paul.

Foulkes, S. H. (1964) *Therapeutic Group Analysis*, London: Allen & Unwin, 1984.

Hobson, R. F. (1979) 'The Messianic community', in R. D. Hinshelwood and N. Manning (eds) *Therapeutic Communities*, London: Routledge & Kegan Paul.

Holden, S. (1990) 'Moving together – the group finds a dance', *Group Analysis* 23 (3): 265–76.

Kohut, H. (1966) 'Forms and transformations of narcicissm', *Journal of American Psychoanalytic Association* 14: 243–77.

Laing, R. D. (1976) *The Facts of Life*, London: Penguin, p. 27.

Levy, F. (1988) *Dance-Movement Therapy – A Healing Art*, Virginia: The American Alliance for Health, PE, Recreation and Dance, pp. 205–19.

Schilder, P. (1950) *The Image and Appearance of the Human Body*, New York: International Universities Press.

Spencer, P. (1985) *Society and the Dance*, Cambridge: Cambridge University Press.

Stern, D. (1985) *The Interpersonal World of the Infant Viewed from Psychoanalysis and Developmental Psychology*, New York: Basic Books.

Taylor, D. and Taylor, J. (1989) *Mental Health in the 1990s*, London: Office of Health Economics.

Tustin, F. (1986) *Autistic Barriers in Neurotic Patients*, London: Karnac Books.

Whyte, R. (1989) 'Symbolism in a group', *British Journal of Psychotherapy* 6(2): 133–42.

Willis, C. (1987) 'Legal and ethical issues of touch in dance movement therapy', *American Journal of Dance Therapy* 10: 41–53.

Winnicott, D. W. (1971) *Playing and Reality*, Harmondsworth, Middx: Penguin, 1982.

Yalom, I. D. (1983) *Inpatient Group Psychotherapy*, New York: Basic Books.

Chapter 8

Individual movement psychotherapy
Dance movement therapy in private practice[1]

Kedzie Penfield

In this chapter I first set out my understanding of movement psychotherapy, then discuss the unique characteristics and techniques of movement and show how they can be used in practice.

INTRODUCTION: THE NATURE OF INDIVIDUAL MOVEMENT PSYCHOTHERAPY

The approach

My work as a psychotherapist is parallel to any other psychotherapy; the common thread is the use of the client's relationship with the therapist to achieve various goals. Although I use words, images, and drawing, my focus is on movement and I use the term 'movement psychotherapy' to describe my work.

I have borrowed from psychotherapy theory, as distinct from the larger field of therapy. My main influence is Irmgard Bartenieff (with Davis, 1965; with Lewis, 1980), whose theoretical and practical skills with Laban Movement Analysis gave me a foundation in a methodology that I treasure. I know of no training other than this American development of Laban's theories that so well emphasizes learning about movement through moving.

Theoretically, I have been influenced by Joan Chodorow (1986), Smallwood (1978), Mary Whitehouse (1977), Harris (1978), Liljan Espenak (1981), and various body therapists including Reich (1969) and Lowen (1967). Of these, private practice is referred to in Chodorow's work, from a Jungian perspective using the Whitehouse authentic movement approach, and by Espenak, although her writing is mainly about hospitalized clients. Espenak's case work is valuable but unfortunately she avoided talking about theoretical constructs and she hardly ever worked verbally.

There is the question of where 'dance' fits into my work. Metaphorically, one can say that any relationship is a dance of one kind or another

– a waltz, a jive, a boxing match to music, or perhaps one person doing a tango whilst desperately trying to relate to a partner who is break-dancing. I use little that is recognizable as 'dance' because I do not choreograph for my clients, or use dance forms or dance steps, and no aspect of performance is emphasized. In an important sense, dance is the ability to symbolize in movement; nobody needs to be a dancer to do that because such dance is neither formalized nor, often, externally visible. The material I work with is usually spontaneous, everyday movement that comes out of walking or gesturing, just as it could be argued that dance itself arises from walking and gesturing. Its discipline requires authenticity and honesty, not technical clarity; 'movement' therefore refers to any action of the body that is actually or potentially communicative, interactive, or expressive.

I work in private practice and also in a social work agency where clients are referred by GPs and social workers. Private clients will have heard about me from friends or participated in one of my workshops and they usually come with past problems, such as abuse of various kinds, or present problems in relationships, particularly with their partners. They may bring fear and a sense of inadequacy, lack of confidence, stress or issues to do with growth, integration, and acceptance of the self. Sometimes it is a fine line between 'healing damage', which is the classic definition of therapy, and 'growth' which is an alternative view. My approach is a combination of these two concepts.

Sometimes I ask people why they believe movement rather than a verbal psychotherapy will help them. They say, 'I've tried vocal therapy and it seems incomplete', or 'well I've always enjoyed moving and words don't seem to get to it for me', or 'I always wanted to use my body to understand myself'. They are all interested in moving rather than just speaking, but are usually articulate people with no resistance to words.

The therapeutic contract

The contract is very individual. It sets the scene and although it changes nine times out of ten – a client begins therapy for one reason, then that reason changes – it is important that the contract is clear. I offer clients a first session without commitment, so that someone can come to find out how I work if they do not already know me. After that we negotiate a contract that includes agreement on issues of payment and time.

The goals and process are discussed. The client's goal might be a happy marriage and three children, and I might suggest that we work with the client's history of relationships with partners; that may not appear to the client to aim directly at the goal. Reaching agreement about the process is therefore very important. For example, one client's goal was about reviewing some childhood experiences but she wanted to work without giving me much verbal information, which is usually acceptable if we are to work through movement. In the first session it became clear to me that the issue was of a childhood experience of sexual abuse. It was extremely damaging to her but had never been identified verbally. By the third session I felt it was necessary to identify the issue, but to do that I needed to renegotiate the contract with the client. We then agreed that the contract should be to look exclusively at her childhood experiences, including verbal sharing of concrete information. However, that really changed the dynamic of the relationship; she had never told anyone the actual facts and my request was as invasive as the original experience. Drawing attention to the contract itself therefore became part of the fabric of the therapeutic process, affecting the rules and the tone.

Once an initial session has led to an agreement to continue I advise a client to commit themselves to six months' work. Many therapists' work is open-ended, but I do this so that clients have no expectation of everything being resolved within two months. Also, by agreeing to work with someone I am committing myself to their process of development; for this, I want the security of knowing that we will work together for at least long enough to discover what might happen. In my experience six months is the minimum amount of time in which this can be assessed.

Therapists are in a position of power, so during the contract there must be constant and careful monitoring of whether they are misusing that power and whether they are working constructively for the benefit of the client. I monitor myself through supervision and I believe that any therapist should do the same to maintain their sense of integrity. The misuse of power is a particular danger in private practice where the therapists have no obligation to talk to anybody about their work, rarely operate as part of a team and are accountable to nobody but the clients themselves.

Supervision is also a support, because a therapist can carry quite a psychic load – the feeling that 'if I have to listen to one more person's problems I will give up'. In movement there may be less verbal disclosure of problems because the work is often on an abstract movement level, but the processes are as strong as in any psychotherapy. Processes like insight, emotional integration, understanding of self, transference, and counter-transference have tremendous power no matter what methods or media are being used.

Although six months is the length of the initial contract, clients usually stay longer, perhaps a year or two. The commitment is likely to be open-ended after six months whether we feel the process has just begun or is about to finish. Towards termination, I will try to make the person more independent, literally aiming at getting them 'on their own feet', and I ask for less concrete information; the aim is to leave the client doing their own work.

The classical psychotherapy model is of one-third of the time is getting to know each other, one-third work, and one-third termination. My norm is a fifth of the time for termination, but however closure is done and however long it takes it needs to happen, just as each session needs its own completion. I have been lucky enough not to have a client storm out on me; there has been some rounding off even with people who have left or people with whom I have refused to work. In fact for me, ending is more difficult than beginning and it often involves an intangible feeling of completing a journey together. Some people then go from being a client to being a supervisee; some ask to come back for an intensive weekend. My intention is that any client will continue their process independently, according to their ability and opportunity.

Summary

To summarize, my approach is probably parallel to that of any other psychotherapist in private practice. I believe the therapeutic process is essentially about the integration, not just the ventilation, of past experiences through the dynamics of the relationship between the client and the therapist; the contract set up between those two people provides the context for integration. Supervision should be used by the therapist to monitor the stresses and dynamics of the working process; then the delicate, invisible magic of psychotherapy can begin no matter what techniques are used.

CHARACTERISTICS OF DANCE MOVEMENT THERAPY

Movement work has certain characteristics that are different from verbal psychotherapy. Movement is another dimension; it can aid learning in a way that words cannot. For some people, including me, words simply do a different job with a different quality.

The seven main characteristics of movement are set out in Table 8.1 and discussed below.

(a) Clarification

The act of talking with someone about a problem can clarify that problem and the situation. Movement clarifies in a totally different way by giving different information. Take anger: one can explore it in movement and see that anger makes one person very tight and rigid and immobilized, makes another person violent and flailing, and

Table 8.1 Characteristics of movement

(a) Clarification
(b) Direct access to the unconscious
(c) Kinaesthetic memory
(d) Simultaneity
(e) Transmutation
(f) Catharsis
(g) Integration

reduces another to using their hands in a very disconnected way. So the movement gives a very individual character to that anger, which clarifies the dynamic of the emotion for that individual. This is different from, not better or worse than, words.

Movement can clarify issues as well as emotion. For example, I once counselled a colleague of mine who is a dancer (this was not therapy) on some major professional choices she was facing. She made symbolic gestures in two directions; one symbolized choreography and teaching, the other represented performing. She improvised with those two different movement ideas, and one allowed her to expand whilst, the other looked more and more damaging to her body. By attending to and following her kinaesthetic movement impulses she allowed her unconscious to 'give its opinion', so to speak, about an apparently intellectual decision. Using words – like 'fragmentation' versus 'focus' – would not, I believe, have given her the same information.

(b) Direct access to the unconscious

A second characteristic is that movement gives direct access to the unconscious. We express ourselves unconsciously through movement but words operate differently; they entail an intellectual process, which movement does not have to do. Words can describe a dream, a movement, an image, or a relationship but they are further removed from the unconscious processes themselves.

The idea that 'the body and its movement cannot lie' is not new. Research and writing about this in DMT includes work by 'Authentic Movement' practitioners such as Janet Adler, Joan Chodorow (1986), and Mary Whitehouse (1977); their Jungian approach includes the concept of 'archetypal movement'. Movement Analysts such as Martha Davis (1970, 1977) and Irmgard Bartinieff (1965, 1980) have developed methods for recording and identifying movement characteristics. In addition, non-verbal communication researchers such as Kendon (1972), Condon (1969), Kestenberg (1975), and Birdwhistell (1970) have given us 'spectacles' through which to observe movement more astutely.

(c) Kinaesthetic memory

A characteristic of movement in general and of bodies in particular is that we have what I call 'kinaesthetic memory'. For example, we all recognize gestures of our own that we acquired from our parents. The musculature of a person who has been hit repeatedly as a child will remember that abuse, even if it is kept from consciousness. All memories, significant and insignificant, are represented in the body, therefore one can access those memories through body or movement work.

I would also argue that the idea that body process is in some sense an inferior process compared to, say, a purely verbal approach, or that it occupies a more lowly rank in the cognitive and intellectual development of the person, is not sustainable. Kinaesthetic memory is as active and fresh a representation of experience as verbal memory because at any point in time, and throughout any experience, one's body is present. If it is active in the experience itself, it can be active not only in the recall but also in the resolution of that experience.

Many techniques of body therapy, which make use of this concept of kinaesthetic memory, are based on the work of Reich (1969) and Lowen (1967).

(d) Simultaneity

Working verbally, a word or sentence must be used for each idea. One word can, but usually does not, encapsulate several ideas; however, one posture or movement can encapsulate three or four.

For example, I remember one client's movement that encapsulated three complex ideas. Her fist came down across her body, really punching at the space, and the word that came to her mind was 'anger'. She also thought of the words 'protective' and 'meditative'. How she got all three of those very diverse ideas into one movement I could not say, but those did turn out to be the processes she wanted to look at and which had to be teased out. Also, as in this example, one movement can encapsulate ideas on different levels of being, such as the emotional, metaphysical, and spiritual.

(e) Transmutation

The fifth idea is what I call transmutation, a 'flip' characteristic of movement. For example, in a stamping dance of anger the movement is furious but suddenly it may transmute or transform; the stamping becomes leaping for joy, so that there is a clear 'flip' from the initial

,emotional state to its opposite. Stamping with anger and jumping for joy involve the same movement; it can also happen, for example, with an embracing movement that suddenly becomes self-protective or comforting. The shape and the energy with which the movement is done are the same but the emotion does a complete about-face.

This is very important in the therapy process because it means the organism is moving, that there is enough health and mobility for the person not to be stuck in one place and so the movement itself generates the flip in a healthy way. Liljan Espenak (1981) does refer to this, although she simply observes the phenomenon and the relationship between jumping and the emotions of anger and joy; transmutation is my own term.

(f) Catharsis

Catharsis refers to tension release of any kind, whether it is anger or fear or joy or love. DMT has a particular contribution to make here because movement is about the physical self and catharsis is a physical discharge of emotion or energy. Other therapies and methods may stimulate catharsis, but it is something that has been borrowed from movement work.

There is a danger that catharsis is seen as the ultimate goal of therapy; that ventilating emotion can expunge it. Ventilation must, I believe, lead to integration, and I treat catharsis as a stepping-stone on the path to healthy integration.

(g) Integration

The seventh and last characteristic is the unique way that movement integrates a process. For instance, a client was working on a bereavement process and had talked a great deal about the loss. She had lost her mother, with whom she'd had a very symbiotic relationship, and although verbal therapy had been completed she came to me asking to work it through in a different way because she felt dissatisfied. On a conscious level she had come to terms with the experience; she knew what it involved and she knew its dynamics, but it had not become integrated at a deeper level.

The climax of our process together was a movement I would call a dance, although it did not look like a dance; it was a movement sequence through which she symbolized a funeral. The movement process, which we did not discuss, was a very powerful thing, almost a ritual. I cannot describe the integration she achieved other than by saying that the loss of her mother was no longer just a loss but had enriched her as a person. The loss would always be there but it was no longer a damaging loss; it was an integrated experience that gave her a deeper appreciation of herself, her mother, and her friends.

TECHNIQUES

Dance movement therapy uses many non-verbal communication techniques borrowed from artistic and therapeutic fields. The techniques I use are numerous, so here I have included only those that are more or less exclusively developed from movement analysis, dance, drama, and Gestalt therapy.

They are grouped into five categories – touch, mirroring, exaggeration, improvisation, and organized movement sequences – which correspond loosely to the developmental stages of childhood, as shown in Table 8.2. Although these techniques can be described separately, often more than one is used at a time just as several movement characteristics can appear simultaneously. Developmental processes also overlap and coexist, combining in new ways, and improvisation enables qualities and kinaesthetic memories to integrate into organized movement sequences.

Table 8.2 Techniques and their developmental parallels

Working method (technique)	Developmental parallel
Touch	First parent/child interaction
Mirroring	Mother reflecting child's movements, facial expression, etc.
Exaggeration	Peer group play
Improvisation	Learning group games, making own rules
Organized movement sequences	Intellectual process of forming a statement

(a) Touch

Touch is probably used more in DMT than in other therapies purposely to develop the therapeutic relationship. The body, when touched, reacts; it cannot remain neutral or literally 'untouched' by the experience in a normally aware, functioning person. There will be a feeling of interaction even with relatively superficial, social contact such as a handshake or a touch on the shoulder.

Touching with a therapeutic purpose falls into two categories, comfort and provocation. Comforting contact is usually from the therapist to the client, or between clients in a group. It often takes the form of a hug or embrace, and can support as well as comfort. For example, I might put my arms around someone standing in front of me, first to comfort them and then to enable them to take a few steps forward with my body strength behind them. Comforting touch affirms both the client and my presence, and has a parallel with a parent–child interaction.

Alternatively, the therapist may consciously use touch to provoke interaction or to work on a client's 'body block'; what is provoked is emotional material. Interactive provocation could include pushing and pulling, or setting up fight structures where the client must break free from being restrained physically, or is invited to push a resistant body away. I explain the structure to the client before it begins so that the provocation is expected, and I often encourage the client to support the exertion with a sound or yell, using phrases such as 'go away!' or 'I won't!'.

The quality of the provocative touch also has an impact on the process; a strong, sustained quality has more control than a quick touch, or one that changes from quick to sustained and strong to light. A light, quick, poking action can be as provocative as a strong movement according to the situation and the body parts used. I remember working with a client whose violent outbursts frequently harmed her children. I wanted her to be able to grade her ability to hit; she seemed to have only an 'on/off' switch rather than the normal ability to express anger with shouting and a violent gesture that harms nobody. I held my palm up in front of her and asked her to slap it. After one slap she could not proceed because the quickness with which I was asking her to clap my hand with hers was too reminiscent of the movements in her outbursts.

We had to find other ways for her to familiarize herself with, and ultimately control, her quick, strong movement impulses. When the quality of our contact changed to a sustained push she began to modify her strength; then with a variety of pushing exercises we worked up to the variations in speed that would simulate her violent episodes. As she became more familiar with and appreciative of the physical sensation of her body when exerting strength, she learned to control the violence and frequency of her episodes.

The developmental parallel is between touch and a human being's first phase of life. Touch is the infant's first contact with the world and, usually through the mother, touch informs the infant of love, protection, and boundaries (Montague 1971). With adult clients these elements are often present, especially when establishing contact. However, some clients do not tolerate touch of any kind, so other techniques must be used for the process agreed in the contract.

Touch can also enhance transference and counter-transference by eliciting it more quickly and more frequently than if physical distance were maintained. With comforting contact, the good parent is present;

similarly, with provocative types of touch, negative transference can more immediately be developed than through verbal interaction alone.

(b) Mirroring

Mirroring is a technique used in dramatherapy as well as in DMT. It usually consists of one person standing in front of another, imitating their movements as if one were their mirror image. The pure version of this technique is done without touching, and it demands considerable concentration from both participants. Variations can include reflection from the side or in a diagonal relationship to the client.

The purpose in all cases is to set up a movement dialogue with the other person. It often leads to other forms of improvisation (see (d) below) but it always makes contact with clients through reflecting their movement. Issues that can be addressed with this technique include the experience of being a leader or follower, and it can be the starting point for tremendous playfulness or a deadly serious interaction.

The more playful aspect of the structure is parallel to a mother reflecting her child's movements. As soon as the first smile appears on the face of an infant, usually at four to six weeks, a mother will respond by imitating the expression. Later, other facial expressions, gestures and vocal sounds are mirrored.

(c) Exaggeration

Exaggeration is a simple technique, also found in Gestalt therapy, consisting of exaggerating someone's movement. For example, if a client does a small tapping of the hand, the therapist might increase the range and intensity by making the hand into a pounding fist. At some point the client will then take over and continue the movement to see where it leads, which will clarify it. The therapist may ask the client whether the movement is about, for example, hitting, comforting, or pushing.

With exaggeration, the developmental parallel is the peer-group play stage. This is what children do on playgrounds – one will do something and another will imitate that action, making it larger and sometimes changing it into something else.

(d) Improvisation

Group play is part of, and leads to, the next technique, improvisation, because developmentally this relates to making up games and rules. Improvisation is a structure that is made up on the spur of the moment to meet the need of the moment. One type is body level improvisation, where for example I see someone moving with very hunched shoulders and I give them a game to play with their shoulders, like making one taller than the other and starting a movement dialogue between the two. Another type is interactive; I could represent a dynamic of their life in movement and they would have to catch me. I remember using that structure with someone who was working on the excessive demands of people and activities in her life, so I poked and pulled at her from many different sides to symbolize the quality of the problems she was experiencing.

Improvisation might take a movement and play with it to see how it develops. Often I will have a sense of the movement someone needs to explore, even if they have not made that movement themselves. Usually clients take the movement I give or reflect back to them and it turns out to be exactly right for some inner process. Playing with the movement may lead to some of the processes described above, like integration or a greater understanding of the self.

Not all clients can participate in improvisation at first. Sometimes I have to spend the first month developing self-confidence, particularly if the client has not moved very much before or has only danced in choreographed movements. People develop the ability to feel comfortable doing 'silly' things, like standing still and listening to their bodies.

(e) Organized movement sequences

The final technique involves forming movement sequences drawn from emotional material, previous interactive structures, body sensations, dreams, or memories. The developmental parallel here is with making an intellectual statement, and the technique is a more complex form of improvisation.

The client is asked to capture and express the memory or body sensation in a movement sequence which is repeatable and visible. How someone choreographs their inner movement into a visible form is uniquely indicative of their inner processes, which are only poorly articulated through words. Is a client's blind rage hitting out anywhere? Is it embedded and carried like a heavy load in the shoulders? Is there a sudden explosion or a slow wind-up of energy which is released only eventually through facial expression or body tension? Although one can generalize that anger, for example, may be expressed through stamping, or misery through holding oneself, the qualities with which these 'personal dances' are done are as important as the actions themselves.

I use this technique often as a closing process for an intensive weekend of work by asking participants to do a 'movement overview' of their experience which they can repeat and show to a partner or to the group. Invariably the sequence that the person shows embodies a process, specific points of experience and personal symbols.

One client was caught in what appeared to be an unbearable situation. He had separated from his wife who had taken their only child, an 11-year-old boy, with her. Two years later he was caught between fury, passivity, and reasonableness. These three states were expressed respectively by hurling himself violently against a wall; sitting cross-legged with a blank expression on his face; and sitting whilst speaking with understanding and patience about his frustration. At one point during our work he did an extraordinary movement, a sustained, strong writhing motion that engaged all his body parts in a three-dimensional, complex form I had never seen before. Desperation, containment, strength, love, and rage were all expressed in this one movement sequence. He looked like a powerful spider caught in his own web.

When he had completed it, his face was fresh and warm; he said he felt liberated. In my perception he had embodied, and therefore integrated, a positive statement of where he was at that moment – in other words, a healthy aspect of his psyche directly expressed the state of his unconscious through movement. To do this he had used the techniques of improvisation and organized movement sequences to allow the power of his body action to further his growth. All seven characteristics of movement had been involved and as a result he felt himself to be a fuller, more actualized person. He had moved away from the place in which he had been stuck, still without solutions to his problem but now able to continue his life with new resources.

CASE ILLUSTRATION – MARGARET

This case illustrates the main characteristics and techniques of DMT described above. I have selected the case because of the specificity of the movement input; it is also an example of DMT used as treatment within the National Health system, where more classical methods are usually employed. The rules of the therapeutic relationship and the characteristics and techniques are the same as in my individual psychotherapy work.

Meeting the client

Margaret was referred by her GP. She was agoraphobic and wouldn't leave her house most of the day; she said very little and she had made a suicide attempt. She was about 35 years old, married with young sons, and had no previous history of depression although her family described her as often quiet and morose. She saw the GP and me alternately, once a week each on different days, and did most of the verbal work with the GP. I talked with the GP every third week about our progress.

I was presented to Margaret as someone who was a movement or physiotherapy specialist. The reason given for me seeing her was so that she could have 'some special time for herself'. She also had tremendous neck pains, which I could work on through massage.

The sessions took place in Margaret's home. She was a small-boned, thin woman of medium height with mousy short hair, always very neatly dressed in muted colours. When she spoke, which was seldom and only when she had to respond to a question, it was in a quiet, metallic voice. I began by massaging her neck for a quarter of an hour whilst she sat in front of me looking out onto her neat garden. I then asked her to move in various ways, rolling her head and reaching in different directions. Finally I asked her to stand up and step forward then sit back down without tightening her neck. She could not do these last actions; she would scrunch her shoulders up, retreat with her head, and heave herself up from her chair. I left the first session feeling that I had established contact with her and the beginning of some trust. I was not sure what sort of language we would have in common.

Margaret's movement characteristics

Margaret's body attitude, as we call it, the posture to which her body habitually returned, was 'fragile vertical'. She carried herself carefully, almost placing herself through her environment, a quality we call 'Bound Flow'. She gave the impression of being able to stop instantly, at any moment, because her movement was so controlled. She even controlled her breathing. Flow is interpreted as the emotional side of an individual, so with depressed patients in particular there is a turning-in of the self, a slowing or deadening of feelings. Reversing that process can result in tremendous anger or sadness. I encourage this reversal; after emotional expression through movement there is always a feeling of relief and an insight. If the flow of an action can be reversed from inward to outward in most cases of depression, a more healthy individual can emerge.

The Bound Flow contributed to her body parts being held in a static relationship to each other, in the same way that her head and neck were in a rigid relationship to her torso. Also, she seemed not to have any personal space at all. Whether we use a large kinesphere – a personal bubble – with our gestures or a small one is determined to some degree by culture and circumstance. When she used gestures, which was seldom, it was usually by poking one body part through her space. The gesture did not support her verbal statement expressively, it just went along for the ride, so to speak.

My overall picture was of a woman who was not in her body; I had the impression that she carried it around as an empty suitcase or envelope and I felt she had no resilience, no ability to adapt to stress in her environment. The other feeling was of the whole of her as a rigidly held container. Her posture and gestures were always very separate. Even when she moved her whole body it was like a gesture of her torso rather than a postural movement or a statement of an involved person.

My working approach began on a body level, simply to give her a sense of being physically present and to educate her kinaesthetic senses. I also wanted to start releasing the control of her flow, allowing her to experience more ease of movement. I intended to use a pushing action to activate her sense of body weight or assertion of self – the two go together and either aspect could be approached first. With a firmer sense of body weight she would feel safe enough to let go some of her rigid control, which was preventing a healthy resilience and adaptability to her life; or with greater ease of movement and sense of being in her own space her use of body weight would come of its own accord. This would also have an organizing effect on other aspects of her movement; posture and gesture would automatically become more balanced.

Finally, I wanted to work on what I called her fragile vertical body attitude. I hoped to help her develop a sense of standing in or moving through her space with a more resilient verticality. Affirming herself spatially as a vertical being was as important as affirming herself dynamically as a strong, present being.

Treatment: the first four months

We began each session with neck massage. There were several reasons for this; it addressed the physical problem for which, in part, she had been referred to me; it allowed me to touch her, so I could start to develop trust and a relationship with her; it addressed the body level pain she had; and it provided a ritual at the beginning of our sessions. It also gave space for the whole aspect of touch referred to above. Other activities in the first four sessions included ordinary everyday movements, level changes, shifting weight, and reaching around trying to make her kinesphere more alive and more available to her.

She did all the actions politely, almost mechanically, with little investment or postural support. In the sixth session she seemed to relax more under my hand and began talking about her childhood, apparently for no particular reason. I stood behind her to do the massage as usual and she spoke simply about her mother's illness, which demanded her assistance and meant taking responsibility for the house and family at an early age. She spoke without ever losing control, giving me new information in an almost meditative way.

I simply listened; she knew I saw the GP and that this would be passed onto him. After the massage I suggested she do the standing sequence again, asking her to allow her breath to support her with a strong exhalation at the moment of shifting her weight up and forward. Gradually we developed this into a strong hiss, rather like an angry snake, she said. I agreed with her image and reaffirmed the strength and flow with which we had done the action. The movement now had a logic, a continuity, a rhythm which made sense and looked comfortable and integrated. I complimented her on her house and garden, encouraging her to take pleasure in the accomplishments of her efforts there. She gave no verbal response to my observation, but seemed to be listening.

She reported to her GP in her verbal session two days later that she had had the first argument in five years with her husband. I did not know the content of the argument but felt that this was a healthy first step in reversing the direction of her destructive energy – from going inwards to herself to going outwards into her environment, parallel, in fact, to the standing up sequence we had been practising.

In our next session she expressed dissatisfaction with her children – she clearly felt guilty about her negative emotions towards them. I accepted what she told me and we worked out other ways of standing, and some walking level changes. I asked her if she had any music she liked that we could improvise to, but she said she had none; she felt silly dancing around to music.

I then asked her to lie on the floor as I wanted to teach her some sequences lying on her back. This was a risk. If someone is flat on their back, with you sitting next to them, there is a danger of them feeling helpless and vulnerable and regressing into unhelpful emotional states. If she had felt too vulnerable her body might have clamped down into numbness. However, the aim was to enlarge the movement sequence of standing up and taking her perceptions out into her life rather than delving down inside herself. I wanted to build up the process of being able to shift spatial levels so that she acquired the flexibility and strength to begin helplessly on the floor, where symbolically she felt she was for much of the time, then stand up in the assertive, clear way we had developed. I was enlarging on this, gradually letting a more sequenced flow arrange her body parts; they would begin to have a smooth progression, a logic, rather than moving in a disconnected way.

At the end of this session she said rather amusingly, 'my husband asked me yesterday what we did in our meetings and I couldn't tell him, except that I enjoy it'. She admitted she felt better after our sessions but did not know why. I took this as a statement of trust and an affirmation that we had reached one of the first stages of therapy, in which a private language is established between patient and therapist. She was beginning to lose the quality of fragility that she usually emanated.

The next sessions continued similarly. I added what I call 'sensing a feeling', which means making distinctions like 'this body sense feels strong, this one feels weak; I like this one, I do not like that one'. I wanted to give her a safe way to begin identifying her emotional self, since this had been deadened in her depressive state. She never expressed strong emotion but she did agree that some body parts were better for her, more comfortable and even more self-affirming than others. She particularly disliked standing up in what she called an awkward way. I encouraged her statements of like and dislike because this kind of statement was about, and from, herself to the world. Her new ability to differentiate between good and bad ways of doing a movement was addressing the aim of appreciating the body itself and contributed to the flow of action in the functional movements of her everyday life.

In her verbal sessions with the doctor she now spoke more aggressively of her life and the complaints she had against her children. She started attending interesting classes outside her home; for example, she asked me if she should try yoga, and she became involved in the local Meals on Wheels programme. She had begun to ask me why we did certain things and if she could work on her own on some sequences, which I encouraged. Her medication was changed and slightly reduced. After the twelfth session, four months from the start of the work, we had a long Christmas break of six weeks.

Treatment: after Christmas

When we began again in February, Margaret had lost some of the vitality she seemed to have gained in our sessions. Christmas had not been joyful; family tension was high and she felt tired most of the time. I tried some of the sequences we had developed for her to practise on her own. She said she had given up after the first week, and now those sequences felt arbitrary and empty. She did what I asked but she was lethargic and uninterested, and whilst her movements did not have the same mechanical quality of our first sessions her curiosity about our work had gone. Her weight quality had become more neutral and her flow more even. I left this session feeling depressed myself. Even the neck massage, with which I had tried to re-establish contact, had felt routine and unsatisfactory.

The next sessions were similar, although she did seem pleased that I came every week. It was decided not to change her medication and that I should see her twice a week. By now her husband was not joining in the couple sessions with what he considered to be 'fake doctors'; he said it was unnecessary and he was very busy. However, this doubling of my sessions lasted only three weeks as things moved very quickly to a conclusion.

The eighteenth session was the turning point of Margaret's process. When I entered she sat down on the couch, said she didn't want to move, didn't want the massage, and didn't want to talk. She neither asked me to leave nor sat passively; she was simply very still. I waited, I suppose about five minutes. Then she looked at me and said quietly, 'What would you say if I told you I was going to kill myself?'

In this instance I felt it was important that she take control of her own process. I acknowledged her statement and waited. She was quiet for a while longer, then asked me if we could do the simplest of movement sequences, standing up by pressing into the ground with bent knees. We did this a few times, then she seemed satisfied and said that was all she needed for that day so I returned to the hospital and told the GP what had happened. He had a session planned with Margaret the next day, so we decided to take the risk and wait until then to see her.

I do not know the content of that verbal session, but after it Margaret was ready to say goodbye to me. In all I had four more sessions with her, during which time her medication was withdrawn completely. She asked me to write down the exercises and tape my voice talking her through our movement sequences. I tried to give her a taste of various physical activities I thought she might enjoy – yoga, 'dancercise', improvisation, and so on – so that she would not feel so unfamiliar and shy if she joined a class. I also asked if she had a friend who could join us so that when I left there would be someone to accompany her in the exercises. None of this worked. She seemed content to take my tape and her notes, as I had asked her to write the sequences down in her own way.

After our twenty-third session and seven months of work I wished her luck, said she could contact me through the health work agency whenever she wished, and then walked out of the door. I never heard from her again. The GP had two more sessions, one with Margaret alone and one with her and her husband, and they both felt we were no longer needed. The treatment goals had been attained – Margaret was no longer on medication, her movement profile was very different, and of her own accord she had said she did not need me any longer – but it was an abrupt conclusion.

Afterthoughts

The main aim for me had been to enable Margaret to stand up on her own, and I felt I managed to do that through her willingness to work in movement. She asked for the conclusion; my personal preference would have been to have a transition into a support system in the community, but given the way I was working the GP did not see any reason to continue and neither did she. I did not have much power to insist. I often want to make sure there are enough supports for the client to continue to grow after we finish. For instance, if a woman has come originally because her relationships with men are unsatisfactory I will expect some resolution of that issue to have taken place, and also a healthy support system to be set up. This may not necessarily mean the development of a wonderful relationship but there should at least be contact with other people with whom the client could talk about the problem.

Usually I set up the support system through the client. I am perfectly open about wanting this network and I will simply suggest that they join this activity or contact these people or engage in this course, or do something that I perceive as supporting indirectly whatever we have worked on. In Margaret's case I suggested attending a yoga class with a friend and continuing her involvement with community activities such as Meals on Wheels. As far as I know, at this point – five years later – she has not been referred again and because she defined her sense of self she is continuing her life as a wife, mother, and person.

CONCLUSION

As in the rest of our lives, a therapist operates in the context of a client's world. In the case study above, Margaret could grow only so far as her world – especially her husband, as well as the culture in which they lived – could tolerate.

The therapist's context is equally important. The experiences, training, supervision, and belief system of the therapist will direct and influence the therapy process. DMT as I practise it is relationship-based work so the people involved are of primary importance to the process. It follows that I cannot work with everyone and that movement is not the best way for every client – psychotherapeutic processes can take place through many different methodologies and techniques.

I do believe, however, that movement has a unique contribution to make to psychotherapy. Through movement we can often understand therapeutic processes differently from the way we can through other methods. Most people need several avenues of approach to clarify their inner journey and growth processes; for many, DMT can be valuable. As Descartes wrote, many years before any of this was conceived of: 'Notre nature est dans le mouvement' (Our nature lies in movement). I would like to paraphrase this to read: *One possibility for growth lies in our body and its movement*.

NOTE

1 This chapter has been edited by Paul Tosey from an interview with Kedzie Penfield.

REFERENCES

Bartenieff, I. and Davis, M. (1965) 'Effort-shape analysis of movement: the unity of expression and function', in M. Davis (ed.) (1972) *Research Approaches to Movement and Personality*, New York: Arno Press.

Bartenieff, I. and Lewis, D. (1980) *Body Movement: Coping with the Environment*, London: Gordon & Breach.

Birdwhistell, R. (1970) *Kinesics and Context*, Philadelphia: University of Pennsylvania Press.

Chodorow, J. (1986) 'The body as symbol: dance movement in analysis', in N. Schwartz-Salant and M. Stein (eds) *The Body in Analysis*, Wilmette, IL: Chiron.

Condon, W. (1969) 'Linguistic kinesic research and dance therapy', *Proceedings of the Third Annual Conference of the American Dance Therapy Association*.

Davis, M. (1970) 'Characteristics of hospitalized psychiatric patients', *Proceedings of the Fifth Annual Conference of the American Dance Therapy Association*, 23–25 October 1970.

——(1977) *Methods of Perceiving Patterns of Small Group Behaviour*, Dance Notation Bureau Press.

Espenak, L. (1981) *Dance Therapy Theory and Application*, Springfield, IL: Charles Thomas.

Harris, J. (ed.) (1978) 'Conversation with Mary Whitehouse', *American Journal of Dance Therapy* II(2).

Kendon, A. (1972) 'Some relationships between body motion and speech: an analysis of an example', in A. W. Seligman and B. Pope, (eds) *Studies in Dyadic Communication*, Elmsford, NY: Pergamon Press.

Kestenberg, J. (1975) *Children and Parents*, New York: Jason Aronson.

Lowen, A. (1967) *The Betrayal of the Body*, New York: Collier Macmillan.

Montague, A. (1971) *Touching*, New York: Columbia University Press.

Reich, W. (1969) *Character Analysis*, New York: Farrar, Straus & Giroux.

Smallwood, J. (1978) 'Dance therapy and the transcendent function', *American Journal of Dance Therapy* II(1).

Whitehouse, M. (1977) 'The transference and dance therapy', *American Journal of Dance Therapy* I(1).

BIBLIOGRAPHY

Guggenbühl-Craig, A. (1971) *Power in the Helping Professions*, Dallas, Tex.: Spring Publications.

Levy, F. J. (1988) *Dance Movement Therapy: A Healing Art*, The American Alliance for Health, Physical Education, Recreation and Dance.

Lewis, P. (ed.) (1979) *Theoretical Approaches in Dance-Movement Therapy*, Vol. 1, Dubuque, IA: Kendall/Hunt.

——(ed.) (1984) *Theoretical Approaches in Dance-Movement Therapy*, Vol. 2, Dubuque, IA: Kendall/Hunt.

Navarre, D. (1982) 'Posture sharing in dyadic interaction', *American Journal of Dance Therapy* 5: 28–42.

Scheflen, A. (1964) 'The significance of posture in communication systems', *Psychiatry* 26.

Schmais, C. and White, E. (1970) Introduction to dance therapy', *Workshop in Dance Therapy; Its Research Potentials*, New York: Committee on Research in Dance.

Chapter 9

On a Jungian approach to dance movement therapy

Amelie Noack

INTRODUCTION

When I was asked to write my contribution to this book, my response was twofold. On one hand I was excited, glad about the opportunity to write about my work. On the other hand, I was wondering if there was a Jungian perspective on dance movement therapy. People like Mary Stark Whitehouse (1979), Penny Lewis (1984), Carolyn Grant Fay (McNeely 1987), and Joan Chodorow (1984, 1986, 1991) who use dance therapy in connection with Jungian principles work in the USA and I had never met them. In the UK Audrey Wethered has written on her approach as early as 1973.

However, I have run many workshops and worked with some individuals, where appropriate, using this combination of dance movement and Jungian ideas. It has grown out of my own experience, a complex mixture of dance, analysis, and body and movement therapy. The ideas of Jung and his followers provide the concept of the collective unconscious and the archetypes; these I understand as a very valuable background and a valid framework for understanding the underlying patterns in movement. Jung himself had patients who used dance as one of the techniques in the analytical work. As it happens he does not elaborate on it, but only remarks that he treated the dance as any other form of active imagination, a technique which will be described later.

There is some literature, for example, Chodorow (1986), which describes dance and movement as part of the individual analytical process. In her chapter 'The body as symbol: dance/movement in analysis' she gives an outline of developmental stages recognizable in movement. Her model is based mainly on the work of Stewart and Stewart (1981), going back to Jung, Neumann (1959, 1970, 1974, 1988), and Piaget (1962). What we can say is that there are some individual attempts to formulate the connections between Jungian thought and dance movement, but there does not exist (as yet) a coherent Jungian perspective applicable to the field of dance movement therapy. I see my contribution as another attempt at a formulation.

To begin with I will give a brief outline of Jung's theory. I will explain his basic understanding of the psychic system and the components which are part of it. I will also give here a short introduction to what Jung termed the process of individuation, the developmental process of the psyche in the second half of life.

Following the theory I will describe the mythological background of dance. The role of the Muse Terpsichore, 'the one who enjoys dancing', is explained in the historical context of the development of consciousness. However, dance is much older than classical Greece and so I have attempted to trace the origins of dance back to the dawn of history.

At the more overt level we all have knowledge of the ritual and its significance in the animal kingdom, with its structured movements and its consequent importance for the continuance of specific species. Equally, as modern quantum science has demonstrated, even the most minute particles seem to have the most intricate dance and movement, which appears to be essential to their actual being, as described by Gary Zukov (1979) in *The Dancing Wu Li Masters*. Whilst I feel unable to delve too deeply into quantum theory, I make the point purely to demonstrate the universal quality of the harmonious relationship involved in the creative process.

At a time when humanity emerged into first glimpses of consciousness, I find a possibility of relating physical movement to psychic. Thus I understand the archetype as representing the psychic inner functioning, in parallel with physical activity and functioning. In this context I explain a central Jungian concept called 'centroversion'. I also reflect on the practical application of Jungian concepts and give examples from my work.

Theoretical background

It seems a very difficult task to present here an abbreviated form of such an extensive body of theory as Jung's. I decided to select those aspects which I personally consider relevant to working with dance movement. I do hope that my selection can be a beginning of an understanding of analytical psychology for the reader. I also hope that it will provide a deeper understanding of the psychological processes which go along with or are invoked through movement, since in this area Jung's findings have proved the most profitable to me.

One of Jung's main concerns was to make people aware of the reality of the psyche. The world of the psyche is different, but is as real as the physical world and has its own laws and structure. The psyche is the totality of all psychic processes and is in constant dynamic movement. The psyche as a whole is made up of two incongruent components, the conscious and the unconscious, both complementing and compensating each other. The agency which mediates between these two areas is called the ego. The ego in itself contains many of those aspects of which we are aware in our daily life. Jung defines the ego as a complex at the centre of the field of consciousness; it has a composite nature and relates all the different processes of psychic functioning, i.e. emotional, cognitive, behavioural, and imaginative activity, and their contents (Jung 1977d: 323).

The unconscious Jung defines as a mixture of personal and transpersonal aspects (Jacobi 1974). The surface level of the unconscious is the personal unconscious. It contains repressed aspects of the individual's life, i.e. memories which are painful or disturbing, and forgotten aspects which can become conscious if necessary. A deeper level of the unconscious he defines as the collective unconscious, which has been described as the 'unknown matrix from which consciousness emerges' (Fordham 1953: 23). 'Here we find . . . impersonal, universal and fundamental characteristics of humanity' (Jung 1977b: 154), which are of a collective nature, and common to all of humanity. The structural elements of the collective unconscious Jung called archetypes. Archetypes are 'a priori conditioning factors . . . [and] represent a special, psychological instance of the biological pattern of behaviour' (Jung 1984: 149). Jung sees archetypes as the inborn tendency to form conscious images and as psychic correspondents to the instincts on a psychological level. The archetype as such is irrepresentable, but 'it has effects which enable us to visualize it, namely, the archetypal images' (Jung 1977c: 213). To give an example, the archetype of the Great Mother as such we cannot perceive. But we can experience her in her positive aspect, for example, as the good mother and in her negative aspect as the 'witch'. The 'now' of our experience is archetypally based, but 'what' we experience, i.e. the conscious image of the respective archetype, is singular, personal, and individual; it is the personal Gestalt of the transpersonal, which has taken form for this particular individual and has thus become conscious. Archetypes are, according to Jung, the transpersonal factors which direct the history of human development.

In the development of the individual it is the interaction with the environment that leads to the differentiation of consciousness from the unconscious and to the consolidation of the ego as the centre and subject of consciousness. By the means of analysis our ego-consciousness introjects contents of the outer world, and consequently reaches, through synthesis, an objective internal picture of the world.

Jung emphasized that there are different stages in life, which fulfil different functions. Childhood and adolescence stand for the 'morning of life', when ego development takes place. During this process the ego gains relative independence and a sense of its singularity and peculiarity, a stage Jung would compare with 'noon-time'. But Jung's main concern was the second half of life, the 'afternoon', and what he termed the process of individuation.

> Individuation means becoming a single, homogenous being, and, in so far as 'individuality' embraces our innermost, last and incomparable uniqueness, it also implies becoming one's own self. We could therefore translate individuation as 'coming to selfhood' or 'self-realization'.
>
> (Jung 1976: 171)

The whole development however follows a pattern called centroversion, which will be described in its relevance to movement further on. Here it should be enough to say that it describes a circular movement around a centre. At the start of the ontological development the movement concentrates on the ego as the centre: its consolidation and differentiation out of the unconscious is the task of the first half of life; it is an initiation into outer reality and a birth into the world. During the process of individuation in the second half of life the process is reversed. According to Jung it is an initiation into the inner reality of the psyche and a birth out of the world. Here a mature ego performs the movement of centroversion around the new centre of the self. It is a process of conscious reflection of so far unconscious aspects of the personality, aiming at the development of the self and at the integration of the psychic system; it is 'the process of assimilating the unconscious . . . where the centre of the total personality no longer coincides with the ego, but with a point midway between the conscious and the unconscious' (Jung 1977b: 219). Jung called this new centre 'the self'. He compares the self to the sun in our solar system, while the ego would be represented by the planet earth, centring around the sun (Jung 1977b: 236). The self is able to reconnect and reconcile opposites, like the conscious and unconscious, good and evil, and masculine and feminine tendencies in the psyche. The self can be felt in the experience of being one-with-oneself and has been related to the Chinese concept of the Tao. Another symbol for the self would be the Yin–Yang, which depicts the interrelatedness of darkness and light.

The process of individuation goes through several stages which are related to archetypal patterns and images. Jung defined these as the persona, the shadow, anima and animus, and the self.

The persona is the role we play in life. 'Persona' is the Latin word for mask and the word 'person' is derived from it. It depicts our social role, the way we like to be seen, and how we like to present ourselves to others and the world in general. A conventional attitude which we use for many years feels familiar and gives security. Every occupation provides a person with a particular role or image to identify with; the same is valid for social class, a social club, or even a nation. All of them provide rules which help people to perform in an expected way, but on the other hand also give rise to many prejudices, because the persona can become a mask or a facade behind which we hide.

As much as conventional role behaviour provides security, it can become a rigid and limiting structure which prevents a person from expressing her or his real nature. On one hand, we all need to develop a persona which suits our individual needs which allows for free expression in a chosen way as well as providing security and acceptance from the environment. However, since the persona is a collective phenomenon, i.e. the role it stands for might as well be played by somebody else, we need to learn to differentiate ourselves from the persona. When that happens the persona becomes an aspect of the personality which can be used as a connecting link with the world and society, as well as a protective barrier against it, according to the circumstances.

In the way that the persona can function as a connecting link with the outer world, the shadow appears as a first connection with our own subjective inner world. In order to grow psychologically we need to confront the shadow, the 'other side' of us, our dark sister or brother. The shadow appears mostly as a figure of our own sex, but shows qualities and attitudes which we dislike, do not want to know about, or cannot accept. The shadow belongs to the ego like an 'alter ego' and represents the undeveloped and uncivilized side of the individual. It is related to the archetype of the adversary, standing against the person's conscious attitude.

Shadow parts of our own personality we often meet in projections onto others of what to us are unacceptable desires, emotions, or actions. But projections can also represent positive aspects of the personality which cannot be accepted. In the therapeutic work unconscious projections can be made conscious and finally the projections can be withdrawn. When that happens, the split-off parts of our own personality are reclaimed and this is often experienced as a gain and increase in physical and psychical energy. Jung points out 'that we cannot be whole without this negative side, that we have a body which, like all bodies, casts a shadow, and that if we deny this body we cease to be three-dimensional and become flat and without substance' (Jung 1977a: 29).

Further concepts which are important in the process of individuation are animus and anima. To explain them here in any depth would go beyond the scope of this chapter. It should be enough to say here that animus and anima are the functions which connect the conscious to the unconscious parts of the personality. Due to the gender-related socialization process we are all subject to, the original disposition of psychic bisexuality is split. The conscious aspects of a man are primarily masculine, while his feminine aspects are relegated to the unconscious. For a woman it is the other way around, her consciousness portrays her developed femininity, while the masculine aspects remain unconscious. However, the development and establishment of the ego and the encounter with the persona, the shadow, and, respectively, anima or animus, are stages on the way to the self, towards self-realization.

What is important to keep in mind is the fact that the stages described have a positive as well as a negative side. They can inhibit or foster psychological growth. The task of the therapeutic work as I see it is to make the archetypal images conscious and to learn to relate to them. This means being able to differentiate them from each other and between the two sides inherent in each. It also means to be able to differentiate them from the ego, i.e. the conscious part of the personality. The latter is of immense importance in order to avoid identification with the archetypal images. The state of identification with an archetypal image is called 'inflation', because a consciousness identified with the archetype has been blown up out of all human proportions. The person has left the sphere of the personal and is literally flooded by the unconscious. This can be most clearly observed in very disturbed people, who believe they are the Queen or Jesus. Here the person has become fixated into the identification with the archetype of the ruler or the redeemer respectively.

However, if a person manages to avoid the dangers and pitfalls of the process, like the identification just described, or is able to work through them, i.e. to dis-identify from the contents and assimilate them consciously, a change can occur. This change is what I have described earlier as the movement towards a new centre of the total personality, the self. This is the Copernican turning point of individuation.

Even then we have to remember that the self can never be grasped fully by consciousness because 'it transcends our powers of imagination to form a clear picture of what we are as a self, for in this operation the part would have to comprehend the whole' (Jung 1977b: 175). Jung describes the self as being the centre of the psyche and at the same time being the whole of the psyche. The experience of the self, and the ongoing process of self-realization, is the aim of individuation.

I am aware that this has had to be obviously a very short and limited introduction to Jungian theory. The interested reader will find a wealth of further information in Jung's own writings in his collected works and in the many works by modern-day Jungians.

The mythological background to dance

Analytical psychology tends to look at mythology in order to explore the archetypal background of the matter at hand. In Greek mythology the figure to whom the area of dance was assigned is the Muse Terpsichore. Hesiod tells us she is, together with her eight sisters, a daughter of Zeus and Mnemosyne (Kerenyi 1958; Larousse 1968).

The stories about the origins of the Muses vary: some say they were three, others nine, but the above mentioned version by Hesiod was generally accepted. Zeus was asked by the other gods, after the victory of the Olympians over the Titans, to create divinities to celebrate this occasion. For nine nights he shared the bed of the Titaness Mnemosyne, who after a year gave birth to nine daughters, whose only concern was song. These were the Muses, goddesses originally linked like the nymphs with the clear waters of springs and virginity, dancing gracefully and displaying the harmony of their voices in song. They were deities presiding over creative inspiration, poetry, and music. Only later were the different themes and the areas and functions of their art distinguished.

Now Terpsichore became the Muse of the dance and some say she educates the young. What is interesting in the Muses' parentage is the fact that they were created in order to praise and glorify the victory of the Olympians over the first divine race, the Titans. This victory has often been connected with the overthrow of the old Cretan order in the Aegean Sea and the establishment of the patriarchal order of classical Greece, which superseded the former matriarchal structure. This change is also reflected in a new mode of consciousness. Psychologically it is the beginning of modern-day patriarchal consciousness (Neumann 1970) with its division into consciousness and unconsciousness, the development of the ego and its differentiation, the basis of our Western culture. Father of the Muses is the master of the new group of the Olympian gods, Zeus, who strikes with lightning and thunder. Mother is the Titaness Mnemosyne, whose name means memory. The Muses carry both their parents' heritage. They were begotten by Zeus and thus stand for the new creative light of consciousness that shows greater clarity and can fertilize and inspire as well as destroy with its might. They were carried and born by Mnemosyne, one of the older goddesses, and therefore the Muses can remember and hold the old; psychologically this means they have access to the past and to the unconscious and can convey it. But their art also brings 'lesmosyne' to humankind, forgetting of sorrows and the ending of suffering, because lesmosyne or lethe was a spring next to the one called Mnemosyne.

The Muses 'enthuse', i.e. bring forth enthusiasm. The original meaning of the Greek word 'to enthuse' is 'to be inspired by the god'. The Muses bestow their gifts and convey their arts to those who are open to them. Theirs is the celebration of the new world order with its new never-ending possibilities of creative consciousness and their inherent dangers. The inspiration the Muses can convey can be true or false (Kerenyi 1958; Larousse 1968). Since they were also related to the god Apollo, in his aspect as God of Music, they are guardians of the oracle at Delphi. In this context they had the gift of prophecy: they revealed that which is, what will be, and what has been.

Terpsichore is the Muse who enjoys dancing. Her name is a combination of the Greek 'terpsis' meaning entertainment and enjoyment, and 'kore', the maiden or daughter. She is the young feminine which brings joy and pleasure. Those whom she loves are filled with the desire to dance.

Greek mythology shows us the deity, the Muse Terpsichore, responsible for dance. This allows us to draw conclusions and to increase our understanding: dance relates to divine energy. This energy can be received by a human being who is open to and favoured by this divinity.

We do know however that dance is much older than the classical culture of Greece.

THEORETICAL APPLICATIONS

Some origins of dance

Dance as a symbolic action is as old as humankind and has long been used for sacred purposes and in ritual (Wosien 1974). Originally dance was a natural expression of being moved by a transcendental power. Chodorow (1984) points out that dance was in the beginning the sacred language through which we communed and communicated with the vast unknown. I like to go further and say that, in the early stages of the development of humanity, dance, movement, and gesture were probably the language in which we communicated not only with the unknown but also with each other. Long before the development of fixed patterns of steps in ritual, dance was a spontaneous expression of personal experience. The whole range of human feelings in the course of one's life can be put into movement. Before the development and differentiation of language, which made a sophisticated verbal communication possible, I imagine movement, sound, and gesture were used to express and communicate feelings and experiences in a very physical and bodily way to other people. We still have access to it today, as can be observed in any dance performance or when people communicate without knowing each other's verbal language. Bodily communication takes over and we can understand what is going on.

For early humanity body and psyche were not conceived of as different as they are for us. Inner and outer worlds were still closely related. What happened in the outside world was directly and personally connected and evoked deep emotional responses. Consciousness was still dormant and experienced every thing or event as a powerful impact, which, for example, in a storm or the change of seasons might overwhelm or endanger life, since the possibilities of reflection and reasoning were still relatively undeveloped.

To feel the impact of a thunderstorm and the ability to allow this to penetrate one's soul deeply and to stir the inside into movement is at first purely physically sensed mirroring, a merely bodily felt reflection of the outer event.

To imitate outer happenings, which in themselves were experienced as powerful and transpersonal, in order to identify with them and thus make them intelligible can thus be seen as the origin of dance. The active act of imitating the thunderstorm in a dance replaces the involuntary and spontaneous impulse by known action and gives conscious reflection a place, allowing internal images and representations to be formed. The body thus becomes an instrument for the expression of this transpersonal power, it is moved by something else, greater than itself. The person dancing can get in touch with a particular life force, a particular archetype, or a particular god. In the terms of Greek mythology it would here mean that Terpsichore was channelling the energy of her father's thunder and lightning.

Identification and imitation are, psychologically speaking, early mechanisms in the development of consciousness in the individual. The development of dance therefore could be seen as a very early mechanism of humanity recreating events of the outside world in rhythmic play. It would be a phylogenetic attempt to create internal images, developing in this way a consciousness of the inner world of the psyche. The enactment and projection of inner experience in movement and dance into the outside world on the other hand allows for classification and testing of inner images and representations and their validity in the relationship to outer reality.

Both the movements here described in their application to dance on a collective level correspond to the two psychological attitudes of 'introversion' and 'extraversion' described by Jung in his typology (Jung 1976). Extraversion is the outward directed movement of energy going towards an object and is aiming at adaptation to the world. Introversion is the inward directed movement of energy going towards the subject and is aiming at adaptation to the internal world of the psyche and the archetypes. The extravert movement affects and alters the world, the introvert lifts inner values and wisdom into consciousness. The exploration of both these attitudes and the exchange between inner image and outer movement has become one of the main tasks in my work, as will be described later. In addition to the two linear patterns of movement which are directed outwardly and inwardly, we find another pattern, the cyclic movement of rotation. This is the oldest form of dance and is to be found in the historical context of ritual. Ritual and dance ritual were originally always round dances or showed a circular pattern, defining a sacred space. In Jungian terms the sacred space is the 'temenos', the protected precinct, and here transformation can occur. Transformation has been defined as a change on a very deep level and this is the aim of every ritual.

The actual physical circular movement around a centre corresponds to the circumambulatio of alchemy (Jung 1980). The psychological going around is again a much later development of the original physical process. Both activities, the outer physical action of the ritual as well as the internal contemplative act of thought, are movements of going around in circles or in spirals. The movement revolves around a central point and in thus directing energy towards the centre actually defines a centre. It is a sacred act and helps to increase the sense of control and security. Neumann (1970) has described this cyclic or spiral pattern in its psychological relevance. It is directed at the development of the personality and aiming at individuation. In addition to the outward directed extraversion and the inwardly directed introversion the third dimension of centroversion comes into play. According to Neumann centroversion is responsible for the development and the consolidation of the ego and the stablization of consciousness. The ego as the centre of consciousness serves to define identity and to give this identity a sense of continuity.

We have here a psychological explanation for the immense importance of circular ritualistic dance in the life of early humanity. Ego-consciousness was still so underdeveloped that it needed the repeated acting-out of con-centrating, i.e. moving around and towards the centre. If the vision of the centre is not re-enacted continuously a dawning consciousness is threatened by the danger of dissolution from the unconscious inside as well as from the world outside. Envisioning the centre becomes a necessity for survival: 'centroversion expresses a natural and fundamental trend of the human psyche, which is operative from the very beginning and which forms the basis not only of self-preservation, but of self-formation as well' (Neumann 1970: 220).

Groups of people who perform a circular dance or ritual, no matter if they live in the Stone Age or nowadays in an African culture or in a Western city, are acting out centroversion. For early humanity establishing a sense of lasting identity for the group through round dances might well have been a necessity of survival in terms of preservation of the species. The individual Shaman however, the magician and medicine man of the tribe, was already in prehistoric time following the pattern of self-preservation and self-formation when whirling around his own axis in a trance.

In the therapeutic application of dance movement, I believe, the importance and the full psychological understanding of the circular pattern of movement cannot be overestimated. Neumann (1959) equals the rotating movement with the gestation process and the maturation and growth process in life. It is a creative and life-giving movement and process, the result of which is a birth. In the early stages of psychological development the process of centroversion is directing the formation of consciousness and working towards the birth of the ego. If there is enough ego, the aim of the process changes, it is now directed towards a widening of the horizon of consciousness and working towards the birth of the self. This later process is the process of self-formation or self-realization. It is searching for meaning and in con-centrating on meaning is defining and creating meaning. Neumann (1959) describes the different stages of this process as stages of matriarchal consciousness: it starts with conception, following fertilization, which psychologically can be seen as an act of recognition or revelation. It is followed by a long time and space of waiting, in which the fertilized egg can differentiate annd mature. This gestation period is reflected on the psychological level in the mental activity of assimilation: we carry the seed of recognition around with us and in us so that it can grow and develop into understanding. The psychological process therefore resembles pregnancy – the outcome is a birth, the result is the realization of meaning.

Processes understood in this way are transformation processes and are directed by the self. The ego is not active here, but observes, supports, and accompanies the process in a receptive way. While the original process of ego development depicts a progression out of the unconscious, the process now aims at an integration of conscious and unconscious. The active centre is not now the ego, but the new centre of the personality, the self. In working with circular patterns in movement, it might be apparent by now that we have to differentiate between three aspects: the temenos, ego-formation, and self-formation. It is extremely important to differentiate the three in order to use them effectively. Each of them stands for a different aspect of circular movement in a developmental context. The temenos stands for the container and the womb and is prenatal. The ego is the focus of psychological development after birth and works with the container of the person's own body and skin boundary. The self can only come into action after the conscious development of the ego and of a psychological container. This psychological container is the psyche as a whole. It is invisible to the outer eye and can be pictured as a bubble containing the body and the conscious personality. The container is invisible exactly because it is the unconscious and not known. All three aspects and their different psychological implications can be observed in movement.

I would like to give here some examples. The first illustrates that which stands for the positive side of the temenos. This was very appropriately expressed by a woman who was struggling through feelings of not having been protected by mother against her invasive father. She said to me: 'I don't want to know anything about you or your personal life; I don't want anything to intrude into these sessions from the outside; I want them totally safe, perfect, like this . . .' and she drew with her right hand a big circle in the air. The movement of her hand allowed her to experience physically the meaning of the symbol of the circle, which goes further and beyond the mental understanding conveyed by the words. Her hand movement told me what her body already knew: the movement of her hand described the circular container of the temenos. I understand this as an expression for her bodily felt experience of the security she had found in the safe space of the therapeutic relationship; a protective mother–daughter relationship, a prerequisite for her future development, had been established.

The second example refers to the circular movement related to the self (like the Shaman mentioned before). A classic example is the whirling dervishes of the Sufi tradition. They circle around their own axis in a continuous movement in order to draw the energy of the spirit down and within. Receiving the divine energy with one hand and passing it on to the earth with the other, they maintain perfect poise and balance in their still centre, which is in communion with the self.

TECHNIQUES

I would now like to describe some techniques from my work. Some will be examples used in workshops, some from my work with individuals. In the latter I generally leave it up to the patient to suggest movement work. But I usually observe gestures and movements which occur spontaneously during a session to increase my understanding, as in the example of the temenos mentioned above. The workshops however were designed with the main emphasis on the exploration of conscious and unconscious aspects of the psyche through movement and dance. This was because I intended to convey in the workshops an understanding of Jungian concepts through practical experience, together with work on the individual's process.

1 Verbal communication

Since movement processes are basically non-verbal processes, they present us with the problem of having to find a verbal translation in order to communicate the experience to others. Often patients themselves offer verbal statements or explanations, but often they do not. In the latter case, I have to rely on my own perceptions, translations, and interpretations. These I may keep to myself or decide later to explore them with the individual concerned, if that is appropriate. Very often it is better to wait until the patient has found his or her own words for the experience. There are also many situations when the movement experience stands for itself and a verbal explanation or interpretation would possibly have detrimental effects. This, I believe generally applies to movements which impress as having a numinous quality. This numinous quality relates to what I have described as the self. It refers to something sacred and bigger than the personalities involved and is frequently connected with the feeling-tone related to awe. Words are insufficient here and often superfluous, since the experience is one concerning the whole of the person, and in this sense goes beyond words.

2 Drawing

Next to verbal communication the technique I find most useful to explore the meaning of movement is drawing. If one applies movement in connection with drawing, it is possible to create a flow of energy, which connects the extraverted and introverted movements of energy mentioned earlier. Inner and outer worlds are related to each other when an inner image can be put into movement. In return the outer movement can evoke an inner image, which then again can be expressed outside on a piece of paper through drawing. The picture thus created can elicit a new impulse for movement and so on. Inner and outer impulse alternate with each other, spark each other off, and foster in this way the process of psychological development.

3 Active imagination

The interaction between inner image and outer movement is based on a technique which Jung termed 'active imagination'. Active imagination is an 'intense concentration on the background of consciousness' (Jung 1977b: 220). The purpose is to perceive what is happening on this background of consciousness. What is perceived is often an image, but also can take any other form, like a musical theme or a movement configuration. Whatever is perceived is looked at or held in consciousness and alterations are noted. The technique of active imagination can be done 'according to individual taste and talent . . . dramatic, dialetic, visual, acoustic, or in the form of dancing, painting, drawing, or modelling!' (Jung 1977c: 202).

CASE ILLUSTRATIONS

Here are some practical examples. The first is to illustrate the usefulness of the alternation between the two different modes of active imagination. A woman, Marge, felt very low and depressed after an exhausting day. Her body was sensed as stiff and rigid. The image which came up was a barren leafless tree in a bleak wintery landscape. This image was held in consciousness and explored through movement. A very slow and gradual process unfolded. Subtle changes in posture, which were barely visible to the observer outside, related to a conscious sensation of gravity and led to a sense of rootedness in the earth and the sensation of sap rising inside the trunk. Light movements of fingers and arms started and the neck relaxed. A swaying movement of the whole body followed, which suggested to the observer the image of a tree rocked gently by the wind, and this was confirmed later. Her arms started to move up and out and, while still standing on the same spot, her whole body looked open, relaxed, and alive, and a smile appeared on her face. Marge finished by opening her eyes and announced: 'Spring has come.' I understand the process as one where the physical sensation of gravity allowed a sense of being supported and nourished; this in turn allowed an opening for change and resulted finally in a new physical as well as mental attitude. Looking at it on an archetypal level, what could be observed was a change from the negative aspect of the Great Mother, who deprives and starves (the winter), to the positive aspect, which is nourishing and supportive and allows growth (the spring).

But movement does not always loosen and open up; it can work the other way around. This happened to John, who worked with me individually. He wanted to explore through movement the meaning of one of his dreams. He could not really remember the dream apart from a sense of being scared. First he moved tentatively, but freely, searching for the right feeling. He was turning around his own axis in a slow anti-clockwise movement. His movements gradually got slower and smaller. He started hugging himself and turned in on himself even more, clutching his hands tightly around his chest, whilst staring at the ground in front of him. To me he looked more and more paralysed. Finally, he stopped moving altogether and stood there without any motion for a long time. He seemed to have become totally unable to move and unable to express what was going on inside. He had turned everything about him inwardly and was holding it inside, exuding a despairing sense of being lost. I finally decided to gently talk to him and I suggested that he drew what he was holding inside.

After a long time he started to do so and covered the sheet in front of him fully with the black colour he had chosen from the box of pastels. When the last bit of the formerly white paper had turned black, he heaved a deep sigh and the paralysed look in his eyes vanished. He looked up at me and then related to me that he was able to contact during the movement and stillness a feeling of great fear. This in turn led to a memory of an incident, when he was 7 years old and had been locked into a shed by mistake. He had re-experienced a deep sense of abandonment. Now he felt immensely relieved, glad that he didn't need to hold the dreadful feeling inside any more, but had been able to express it and look at it on the outside together with me.

In this context I would like to add another important aspect concerning the direction of movement, which applies to outward and inward directed movement as well as to circular movement. As Jung points out, the direction from left to right is a movement towards consciousness. It is related to progression, while regression relates to the reversed movement of right to left, pointing to the unconscious. It is important to keep in mind that both directions are important and need to be integrated (Jung 1985: 200). Contrary to the common use of right and left, they are not to be understood or used as a value judgement. John's slight left-orientated turning movement is the searching in the unconscious for a content, a feeling, or an explanation, which as a result lends new clarity and insight to consciousness.

As much as we need both introversion and extraversion in order to function fully in life, we need for the same purpose also times of regression and times when we can progress.

Ultimately the goal is the integration of the opposites and the movement which occurs in this respect shows, in my experience, a vertical flow of energy. This can be upward as well as downward directed, depending on the context and the situation. I explored the principle of integration, which is reflected in the upward directed movement, in several workshops, where I used Jung's model of the stages of life in connection with his elaboration of the tree symbolism (Jung 1983). Jung sees the tree as a symbol and model for individuation (see also Mindell 1982). In Marge's case it appeared spontaneously. In the workshops I applied the tree symbolism to movement, interpreting movements in the space close to the ground as belonging and relating to childhood. Close to the ground is where our roots are and we need to have them firmly planted, before we can stand erect. In infancy and babyhood we live and move exclusively near to the ground, unless we are picked up by an adult. I applied this in the workshop and the movements restricted to the area of the ground brought up a lot of unconscious material, which had been found on the floor so to speak, and which related to childhood.

Accordingly, patterns and movements which related to the here and now of adulthood were expressed and explored standing upright. The torso represents the trunk of the tree, the ego, having become differentiated from the unconscious ground. The adult who has developed a mature ego has his or her own conscious standpoint. An adult is able consciously to perceive, realize, influence, and alter things. Movements here often manifest on a horizontal level.

The third area and the third kind of patterns explored were related to the area above and beyond the body, the crown of the tree. This relates to the second half of life and the process of individuation.

The area above and beyond the body is concerned with what and how far we can reach when standing upright on the ground. This reaching up and out is not now for a parental figure or for an adult partner. Only when those needs have been fulfilled satisfactorily can the new pattern develop fully. It can then become a way to reach out for and comprehend the aims and goals of our individual life. The body here needs to be in a firm connection with the ground and with reality, and represents the ego of the adult person, which is striving to reach out and relate to the self.

To use again John's example to illustrate the first and second area of roots and trunk. John was on his feet and standing upright during his exploration. However, his eyes were firmly fixed on the ground, as if he was watching and observing some scene or situation. He could see something down there on the ground, in what I have called the area of childhood. He was able to pick something up from the floor with the help of his eyes. My interpretation is that he was at the same time able to stay consciously in contact with his ego, while exploring and experiencing a childhood situation, which needed to be integrated.

When it is possible to connect these two areas in the therapeutic work as happened with John, an opportunity is provided for the person consciously to connect the adult with the child within. A group participant described this event very movingly as welcoming a little child into his arms.

Another example which illustrates this point connecting it with the developmental process is the case of Nina. When she began working with me, which by now is several years ago, she was very depressed and lived as she said in a black cloud. This related to a very deprived childhood where she received hardly any mothering. When she walked in for her sessions her movements were almost limp, walking seemed hard work, and she looked as if there was no life within her. At the start she used to sit on the couch in a kind of rigid position, hardly moving at all. As time went by she started to relax bit by bit. Often she grabbed a cushion holding it tightly in front of her belly, for protection she said. After about eighteen months she began to pull her feet up and in one session rolled herself up into a foetal position still clasping the cushion, which had become either a nourishing placenta or transitional object. She felt safe, she said, like this and returned to this position regularly over a period of several months. One day she told me a dream, while sitting on the couch. In this dream she was walking down into a narrow passage which turned into a dark tunnel, at the end of which she could see some light. She said in the dream she had experienced a kind of forward-pulling movement which she could feel throughout her whole body. In order to demonstrate this she moved her arms in a swimming stroke forward and downward, repeating it over and over again whilst talking. I brought her attention to her movement and asked her to feel it consciously and follow any intention she could sense in her body. Sitting on the edge of the couch she could begin moving forward and downwards following her arms at first. When her head and shoulders touched the ground her arms stopped guiding and followed behind and alongside the trunk of her body. Slow, twisting and curling movements, beginning at the head, moved throughout her whole body until she was fully lying on the ground. There she stayed for the rest of that session. In response to my question, did she wish to say anything before we finished, she said no, she just wanted to lie there and feel it and continue like this next time.

She did just this, for several sessions, saying she felt much safer on the floor than she ever did on the couch. During this time we discussed her dream as relating to birth, but also to getting in touch with a deeper and darker aspect of herself, which I related to the shadow. It also became clear that the process of moving through the dark tunnel was related to the dark cloud she had felt enveloped by. In the dream and once more during the session she had been able to accept the darkness and move into it and through it.

Nina spent exactly seven sessions lying on the floor and then announced she now felt ready to sit up, which she did, leaning with her back against the couch and facing me. I had been aware that the way she had been entering and leaving the room at the beginning and the end of the session had been slightly different since the tunnel dream. But the process seemed to be completed only now with her sitting up opposite me. When she stood up at the end to walk out she seemed to me more balanced and I felt that for the first time she was using the ground fully. This time it seemed to me it was not her mind dragging her body up from the ground, by will power, but the contrary. Her body was able to use the firmness and resistance of the ground in order to build itself up on top of her feet. This is how I saw it while observing her, but it was confirmed when she came the next time. She told me very excitedly how special walking had felt since she saw me the last time; she had never felt like this before!

I would now like to return to the model of the tree and the movement related to it.

Those movements which relate to the third area of the crown and to individuation, I have termed 'Tai-chi' movements. I have seen it again and again, that a person who succeeds in embodying some sense of the self moves in a very balanced and harmonious way, which is not consciously directed by the ego. The movements are centred, slow, and flowing. There is stillness in the movement, and the movement itself seems to materialize in stillness. Being allowed to watch it feels to me each time like a great privilege.

As Arnold Mindell writes

> The person governed only by time and social pressure is not in contact with the body spirit or the self. . . . The individual who is aware and manifests inner life dances . . . effortlessly.
>
> (Mindell 1982: 23)

The images people have put onto paper after such effortless dance and balanced movement are symbols of the self: the sun, a newborn baby, a bird, golden apples, the tree of life, a star, to name only a few.

The working through of childhood experiences, relating these to the ego and consequently trying to reach further towards individuation, as was possible for some individuals in these workshops, seems to have had the effect of establishing – if only for a short time – what Jung calls the transcendent function. The transcendent function lifts an insoluble conflict above and beyond the area of conflict, in facilitating the union of opposites. In creating a new balance between the ego and the unconscious, it brings about a new attitude (Jung 1977a: 97). This new attitude of contact with the self, I believe, is what can be expressed in the 'Tai-Chi' movements.

CONCLUSIONS

This material has sought to establish a linkage primarily between dance movement therapy and Jung's concept of the psyche and its development. The basic human questions, like: what is the driving force behind movement or action? What is it that sets us in motion? What moves us?, I hope have become more clear. The foetus already moves in the womb. Birth, the process of being born, is first and foremost movement. It occurs at the moment of subtle interaction of inner forces in the baby with the external reality of the womb and its contractions.

Emotion in becoming motion leads to dance and ritual, thus giving external expression to the psychic reality of the archetype.

SUMMARY

In this chapter I have tried to take note of both inner and outer realities. This follows from my belief that one is the mirror of the other and, in order fully to live one's life, these attitudes need to be consciously related to each other. I have attempted to convey a particular understanding of movement and movement processes which I have developed with the help of Jungian ideas and thought.

DMT is such a young field. It is one of the creative techniques of which more and more use is made in therapeutic work. My personal experience, in my own analysis as well as in my therapeutic practice, is that the human being is such a complex creature that therapeutic work is often seen as first and foremost the development of mental representations. I believe this is not the whole story, and perhaps the mental representations are not necessarily always verbal. In therapy we are dealing with the psyche, the psychological world, and I believe this world contains much that is still unexplored and uncharted.

REFERENCES

Chodorow, J. (1984) 'To move and be moved', *Quadrant* 17(2).
——(1986) 'The body as symbol: dance/movement in analysis', in N. Schwartz-Salant and M. Stein (eds) *The Body in Analysis*, Illinois: Chiron.
——(1991) *Dance Therapy and Depth Psychology*, London: Routledge.
Fordham, F. (1953) *An Introduction to Jung's Psychology*, Harmondsworth, Middx: Penguin.
Jacobi, J. (1974) *Complex/Archetype/Symbol*, New York: Princeton University Press
Jung, C. G. (1976) *Psychological Types*, *Collected Works* 6, Princeton: Princeton University Press.
——(1977a) *On the Psychology of the Unconscious*, CW7, London: Routledge & Kegan Paul.
——(1977b) *The Relations between the Ego and the Unconscious*, CW7, London: Routledge & Kegan Paul.
——(1977c) *On the Nature of the Psyche*, CW8, London: Routledge & Kegan Paul.
——(1977d) *Spirit and Life*, CW8, London: Routledge & Kegan Paul.
——(1980) *Psychology and Alchemy*, CW12, London: Routledge & Kegan Paul.
——(1983) *The Philosophical Tree*, CW13, Princeton: Princeton University Press.

——(1984) *A Psychological Approach to the Dogma of the Trinity*, CW11, Princeton: Princeton University Press.

——(1985) *The Psychology of the Transference*, CW16, Princeton: Princeton University Press.

Kerenyi, C. (1958) *The Gods of the Greeks*, Harmondsworth, Middx: Penguin.

Larousse (1968) *New Larousse Encyclopedia of Mythology*, London: Hamlyn.

Lewis, P. (1984) 'Object relations within a Jungian perspective', in P. Lewis (ed.) *Theoretical Approaches in Dance-Movement Therapy*, Vol. 2, Dubuque, IA: Kendall/Hunt.

Lewis, P. and Avstreih, A. (1984) 'Object relations and self psychology within psychoanalytic and Jungian dance-movement therapy', in P. Lewis (ed.) *Theoretical Approaches in Dance-Movement Therapy*, Vol. 2, Dubuque, IA: Kendall/Hunt.

McNeely, D. A. (1987) *Touching*, Toronto: Inner City Books.

Mindell, A. (1982) *Dreambody*, California: Sigo Press.

Neumann, E. (1959) *The Psychological Stages of Feminine Development*, in *Spring*, New York: Psychological Psychology Club.

——(1970) *The Origins and History of Consciousness*, Princeton: Princeton University Press.

——(1974) *The Great Mother*, Princeton: Princeton University Press.

——(1988) *The Child*, London: Karnac.

Piaget, J. (1962) *Play, Dreams and Imitation in Childhood*, New York: Norton.

Stewart, L. H. and Stewart, C. J. (1981) 'Play, games and stages of development', *Proceedings of 7th Conference Association of Anthropological Study of Play*, Fort Worth.

Wethered, A. (1973) *Drama and Movement in Therapy*, London: Macdonald and Evans.

Whitehouse, M. (1979) 'C. G. Jung and dance therapy: two major principles', in P. Lewis (ed.) *Theoretical Approaches in Dance-Movement Therapy*, Vol. 1, Dubuque, IA: Kendall/Hunt.

Wosien, M. (1974) *Sacred Dance*, London: Thames & Hudson.

Zukov, G. (1979) *The Dancing Wu Li Masters*, London: Fontana, 1980.

Chapter 10

Dance? Of course I can!

Dance movement therapy for people with learning difficulties

Jeannette MacDonald

INTRODUCTION

Very little has been written about DMT for people with learning difficulties. I hope that this chapter will redress the balance somewhat by lifting the veil and allowing some of the philosophical, practical, and possibly contentious aspects to be examined. Through my work with this population I have, necessarily, developed theories and strategies which I hope will be of interest, and will enthuse others to step into this particular dance which is often happy, sometimes sad, occasionally frustrating, ladled with humour, and never dull.

It has now become quite acceptable to reject the model of a mind–body dichotomy in favour of a unitary view of the person as a single organism. Events that affect the organism affect the *entire* organism. Anything that affects the body inexorably affects the mind and vice versa. A trained and experienced dancer has an intuitive knowledge of the mind–body continuum. It was from a dancer's perspective that I came to work with this population. Since my early work in 1973 that perspective has broadened and that initial intuitive approach has been sharpened and substantiated. Dance is rhythmic, expressive movement. Some form of dance can be found in every culture and traced back to the dim beginnings of human expression. Without movement there is no life. Movement is one of the criteria for life in any organism. We are surrounded by the rhythms of our natural world and rhythm brings order, for example, the lunar rhythm, the circadian rhythm, or our own bio-rhythms, and because dance *is* rhythmic movement it is a wonderful tool to bring order into disordered lives.

The approach

Who are people with learning difficulties? Apart from the common bond of mental retardation in varying degrees and complexities they are individuals as unique and diverse as the rest of the population. Those with profound learning difficulty may be unable to hear, see, or speak. They may have spastic limbs and limited capacity for movement. Is DMT appropriate for such people? I believe that it is not only appropriate but vital because often the smallest movement, even if it is assisted, affords each individual a window, however small, into their own feelings. This will be seen later when we come to look at specific case studies.

The physical and emotional problems that present under the label 'learning difficulty' run the gamut from mild mental disability and no physical disability to profound mental, physical, and sensory disability. The idea that DMT with this client group is limited and limiting must be firmly laid to rest. The only limitation is that of the individual therapist. There is a constant need to find a new approach – a way around physical limitations – developing dialogues with other disciplines and always dipping deeply into one's own resources. These resources, therefore, must be firmly based. I feel that a strong dance background and knowledge is essential if one is to engage in any meaningful therapy. By dance background I mean training and not simply passive enthusiasm. Only through the physical experience of a movement or gesture can one understand the feeling behind that movement. In therapy it is often necessary to provoke feelings through particular movements or to recognize the feeling behind a movement or series of movements. Without some form of personal dance training this can be very difficult. Since dance focuses on the expressive quality of movement rather than on the movement as an end in itself, I believe that a dance education is preferable to other forms of physical education as a basis for this field of therapy. A dance movement therapist must know personally what it is to dance: why it is difficult, how it becomes easy, and how a particular movement can happen anatomically. This 'knowing' includes an awareness of the effect a movement can have on mood and emotion, and of how connecting certain movements together adds to or diminishes the inner feeling. It includes knowing how it feels to leap into the air, how it feels to know *how* to leap higher, how to syncopate a rhythm – move with a rhythm – against a rhythm and how this *feels*.

A rich vocabulary of dance techniques and cultural forms is an essential resource and should be acquired before contemplating training in DMT. A sound knowledge of human anatomy and physiology is important if one is to work confidently with, for example, people with learning difficulties who may also have a physical disability. An understanding of how each joint works and its normal range of movement is necessary when working with clients with spastic limbs. One often has to move with and for these clients and therefore an understanding of, for example, how much movement to pursue, how far and in which direction is vital in order to avoid pain or confusion for the client and consequently a disinclination to co-operate with the therapist.

In addition, particularly for working with people with learning difficulties, a good knowledge of developmental movement is required. Omitted developmental patterns may have a profound psychological impact. It is also important to be able to focus on the 'child' in oneself, to be able to play without inhibition. Some adults with learning difficulties can be very 'child-like' and one needs the ability to relate at that level without being patronizing. Both Winnicott (1971) and Sutherland (1980) agree with the hypothesis that playing becomes the prototype for the therapy experience with both children and adults. 'It is only in playing that the individual – child or adult – uses his whole personality in creative activity, and it is only in creative activity that he discovers this self' (Sutherland 1980: 852). I have found it necessary to have an eclectic response to a variety of psychotherapeutic theories and practice to meet the needs of individual clients. The work of Jung, Klein, Winnicott, and Bowlby seems to underlie much of my own practice but I would emphasize the necessity of a broad study of psychotherapeutic theory and vigilant questioning and evaluation of one's own work. In order to bind these 'ingredients' and have an appreciation of the therapeutic process one must also undertake one's own therapy.

Physiological and developmental aspects

It would appear that the desire to dance is primitive to the human organism. The majority of normally developing infants usually exhibit this desire to dance once they have achieved an upright stable posture. In the developmental process, in order to reach an upright posture, stand, and then walk, certain primitive postural reflexes must be assimilated and replaced by voluntary motor responses. One important reflex which must be assimilated is the 'tonic labyrinthine reflex'. This is the primitive reflex to the fear of falling and if it has not been assimilated by the onset of walking the infant will exhibit great difficulty in motor control because of dominant flexor patterns. Feldenkrais (1966) claims that this fear of falling is constantly present to some extent in anyone who has not assimilated the tonic labyrinthine reflex. This must severely limit the performance of any activity. Living in a constant state of anxiety necessarily inhibits the desire and motivation to explore and learn in the way of normally developing infants. People with learning difficulties are not developing normally because of some element of brain damage, genetic, chemical, or traumatic. I have frequently observed these dominant flexor patterns and consequent anxieties in many profoundly disabled clients.

In order for the brain to function well it must be able to both *receive* and *process* a constant stream of stimuli, especially from the body. If the brain can develop the ability to receive, remember, and then motor plan, this ability can then be applied to all sorts of activities regardless of the specific content. The early work of Bender and Boas (1941) at Belle Vue Hospital, New York, took a number of schizophrenic children through a varied intensive programme of movement activity – crawling, rolling, jumping, etc., and noted marked changes in their general behaviour and level of functioning, particularly in the areas of responsiveness and attention span. If we examine the 'Sensory Integration' theories from the studies of Lorna Jean King (1974) and Jean Ayres (1975) we see that the tactile, vestibular, and proprioceptive systems are the earliest to mature. The vestibular system orients the body in space and its movements through space. This is intricately linked with muscle tone, balance, oculomotor control, visual and auditory perception, co-ordination, and tactile functions as well as autonomic functions such as heart rate, respiration, vaso-motor functions, and emotions. Figure 10.1 shows how underdevelopment of this system affects cognitive skills and therefore affects learning.

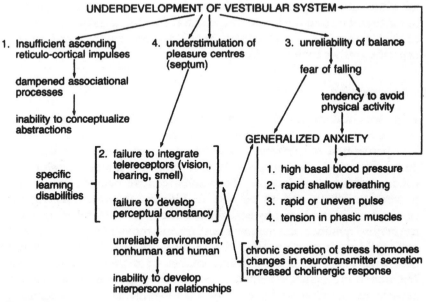

Figure 10.1

These and other studies seem to add weight to my own theory that, especially for people with learning difficulties, it is vital to develop early sensorimotor skills. I have observed clients with learning difficulties, in

OT sessions, successfully complete simple shape discrimination and sequencing boards over and over again and yet the same clients in DMT sessions have been quite unable to discriminate body shape or manipulate small and large balls through graded spaces. Dysfunction shown in postural and bilateral integration suggests that early perceptual skills are not intact. I believe that these clients have simply learnt to manipulate the specific pieces of equipment in their OT sessions successfully, but the learning is superficial – they do not know *how* to use it. It is important that the brain develops the *capacity* to perceive, remember, and motor plan. This ability can then be applied towards the *mastery* of all academic and other tasks regardless of the *specific* content or context. The role of DMT in sensory integration is obvious. Walking, running, jumping, twisting, rolling are all gross motor activities and through the language of dance become expressive and enjoyable rather than mere tedious exercise. Engaging the enthusiasm of those with learning difficulties for an activity is vital as generally their span of concentration tends to be limited and the added dimension of enthusiasm can sometimes extend that span. They enjoy *repeating* movement patterns, however simple. In this way they develop movement memory and gain experience on which they will be able to draw for future activities and accomplishments. The key to development lies in the therapist's ability to *observe* and *assess* the individual's response and to devise a variety of dance movement situations and activities to elicit capacities rather than their incapacities.

TECHNIQUES

What we think of ourselves and what others think of us depends to a large extent on our self-image and the reactions it evokes in others. The perception of physical image has a direct bearing on the inner perception of self. Self-image is an important determinant of behaviour. Clients need to feel that they have some control over the image they present to others and to be able to identify the inner feeling that corresponds with that physical presentation. It is useful to focus on the *positive* qualities of a person's posture and movement; for example, I use a full-length mirror to allow them to observe their capacity to change their own image, to become taller, smaller, or more fierce, gentle, etc. The mirror is a valuable feedback tool in allowing them to observe and experience the effects of their physical movements, and to bring the various parts of their bodies into conscious control.

Many people with learning difficulties have great problems with relating to their own bodies and recognizing body parts. Simple rhythmical dance games can enable them to identify parts of their bodies, relate to them as their own, and experience their capacity to use them in many different ways. Much of this initial work must necessarily be quite didactic and time needs to be spent in providing a movement vocabulary and enabling an acquisition of gross and fine motor skills that are taken for granted when working with other populations. We cannot expect the sort of progress we would see in normally developing children. It is a longer, slower process.

In my experience rhythm is paramount in this early work. It can help the clients to develop a sense of structure and organization in their confused and chaotic private worlds. The continuous basic beat and repetition of a rhythmic structure provides an expectancy that helps to alleviate their fear of the unknown. It can also facilitate physical co-ordination and co-operation with others. Rhythms are energizing and inviting and may stimulate different qualities and patterns for those who might resist spontaneous movement. A waltz rhythm, for example, may stimulate large whole body movements and encourage a broad use of space. Tyrolean slapping and stamping rhythms may promote strong and forceful movements and also may relieve tensions and aggression.

When considering rhythm most people automatically look to music, but often music can be intrusive and distracting. Whilst not suggesting that we should dispense entirely with music I believe that we should be most careful in our choice of it, using it to reinforce a chosen rhythm or to create a particular mood. People made music with their bodies long before they made instruments to play that music. Dance came before music and so for dance movement in therapy I believe we should return to that natural progression.

Many people with learning difficulty have no speech. Not to speak does not mean that one has nothing to say. Those without speech may be bubbling with emotions which can be expressed only in gesture and play of features, sometimes resulting in deep frustration. Movement and gesture are the means of communication for young infants before the development of speech. Self and interactional motor synchrony are precursors to speech in normal infants. Children with learning difficulties show problems in moving synchronously with sound, including human speech. The greater this problem seems to be, the greater the autistic-like isolation from people and the world. Only through a delicate dance of action and reaction between a more experienced and a less experienced human communicator can shared meanings be arrived at. The development of language depends upon the prior development of communication itself. It is clear that the therapist working with clients with learning difficulties, particularly those without speech, needs to develop good personal relationships with them before communication can become positive and meaningful. Dance and mime are natural vehicles for non-verbal communication. Moving together in harmony *is* communication. Many people find that they can express through dance thoughts and emotions for which they have no words, even though they may have speech. Dance and mime activity can obviate much frustration and also act as a safe channel for the release of otherwise unexpressed emotions and ideas.

When I began this work I found myself with very large groups of people with diverse and varying disability. Although it taught me a great deal about leading and managing such groups, inevitably the quality of therapy for the individuals in those groups must have been very limited and afforded little opportunity to develop the strong individual empathy required for meaningful therapy to take place. In fact, one must conclude that such work with large groups is almost always recreational rather than specifically therapeutic regardless of the focus. This is because people with learning difficulties generally have a poor self-image and without some idea of self the benefits of interactional groupwork are very small. The result is that most of my work in this field now is with individuals or with very small groups (no more than four) with similar needs.

When individuals are referred for therapy the reasons stated tend to be broadly along the lines of 'improving posture, gait, body image, etc.', but it is so important to remember that DMT is not simply a physical therapy. I spend most of my first session with individuals chatting over a cup of tea or coffee, drawing or painting, or simply sitting quietly together listening to some music of their choice. This is necessary in order to build some personal empathy before beginning any movement work. Most people have an intuitive knowledge that movement is exposing and they can be, initially, very timid about that 'first move'. It makes them feel vulnerable. They wonder if they are moving 'correctly'. I usually start by suggesting a theme. People like to have a reason to move. Often I take the elements – earth, fire, air, water – and ask them to choose one of these as their theme. So we have a beginning – something to express. I suggest that we move together – inviting – 'Let us' – 'Shall we?' – 'Perhaps we could . . .', showing movement ideas, pathways, rhythms. Then slowly, slowly 'What do you think?', 'How would you do this?', until one is eliciting their own spontaneous movements and gestures. The theme may change, it may become irrelevant. It does not matter. They are moving, by themselves and for themselves. Self is in focus. The theme is a tool.

I do not want to give the impression that this is a facile process. One should not expect it to happen within a couple of sessions. It can take very many sessions over a long period of time and sometimes, even with time, patience, and persistence, the authentic movement does not come. This is an example of working with clients who have reasonable comprehension and physical ability, it cannot be attempted with the more profoundly disabled.

Close physical contact is a good place to begin with the profoundly physically disabled who also have learning difficulties, so that they might experience assisted movement. By this I do not mean frontal body contact, which can be very threatening, but body moulding so that the front of the therapist's body is in contact with the client's back. Sitting or lying on firm quality floor mats, the therapist makes large, slow arm and leg movements, one side of the body, then the other, then bilaterally. Music can be of enormous benefit here to aid rhythm and flow. Continuing in the same way the therapist makes whole body movements, closing tightly and opening at full stretch. Great sensitivity to the client's physical capacity is required throughout this process. It should be totally pleasurable. Any physical discomfort they experience will delay or possibly prevent the building of the personal empathy and trust that is needed to continue. If the therapist is at all unsure they should always seek the advice of other professional colleagues – doctor, physiotherapist, nurse, etc. The client must always be approached with confidence. A sure and confident approach imbues them with a vital feeling of reliance and hope without which one cannot work meaningfully.

'Me' and 'you' can be awkward concepts for clients with learning difficulties. An understanding of these boundaries is essential for good social interaction and there is much movement work which can be used to help them gain this understanding. For example, with a small group of clients we might walk around in the space with eyes cast downwards, making no eye contact. We might make closing gestures towards ourselves, occasionally uttering the word 'me' as we all move at our own speed. Still walking around the space we might begin to look up and make eye contact with one another. We do not stop moving. We start to make opening gestures towards others in the group as we pass, occasionally uttering the word 'you'. We adjust our speed to each other so that eventually we are moving at the same speed. We alternate these movement patterns. Depending on the group this work has a way of developing its own momentum into interesting dance pieces. It can be used as a starting point to develop the concepts of 'self' and 'other' and to integrate inhibited members of the group. Initially the therapist joins in but ultimately steps aside to observe and gain insight into individual difficulties.

We can use body tapping rhythms to help lateral and cross-lateral problems. Clapping a simple rhythm can encourage the client to reproduce it in any way – clapping, stamping, or even vocally. They require plenty of time to establish the rhythm before transferring the clapping to tapping body parts – hands, knees, elbows, head, etc. It could start with one hand tapping one side of the body and then go on to use both sides of the body and both hands for tapping, keeping the rhythm clear and simple. More complex tapping patterns and rhythms can be developed later. This is often great fun with much laughter. It should be kept well within their capacity. These clients know what it is to fail, the therapist needs to help them to succeed.

I believe that therapists need to develop their own techniques so that they are firmly based on personal understanding and therapeutic goals. I hope, therefore, that the techniques illustrated will be used only as starting points or to spark ideas, and not as an end in themselves. It is experience which brings the insights needed to pursue seemingly superficial exercises towards meaningful therapy.

Settings

Where does all this take place? When I first started this work in the early seventies most of those with learning difficulties were in long-stay institutions and special schools. Now many of those institutions are closed or closing and children with learning difficulties are being integrated into mainstream schools or special units attached to them. Adults are being dispersed into hostels, flats, and houses for independent living with minimum supervision or back to their own homes with community team care. Unfortunately, the closing and dispersing seems to have happened, in many places, before adequate community provision is in place. One hopes that this situation will soon be ameliorated, before we have a cry to return to institutional care simply because of a lack of adequate community provision.

When the institutions began closing, a number of creative therapy colleagues and myself persuaded our local health authority to fund a 'Creative Therapy Unit' (art, music, drama, and dance movement therapy) within the community. This finally came into being in late 1985 and is now a generic community resource, the first of its kind within the NHS in the UK. It is this setting in which I have been able to work the most fruitfully and I believe that it is the best model for the creative therapies. I would like to see it adopted in future community developments. I have worked in many settings over the years – schools, hospitals, day centres, clinics, colleges, clients' homes, and in private practice – and ultimately I find that the issue of access is crucial. Only in an open, statutorily funded centre can DMT and the creative therapies generally be accessible to all. Working in a centre with other creative therapists also provides support, feedback, and the peer group supervision necessary to maintain the checks and balances on our work. It can be very isolating work, especially in private practice, and one needs to have a good network of professional colleagues for advice and reassurance in times of difficulty.

Resources

Wherever one works one needs to have a reasonably spacious, un-impeded room with a sound wooden floor or smooth floor covering. It should have good access for wheelchairs, pushchairs, etc., and some degree of privacy. These are basic essentials. I also like to have:

1 a full-length mirror;
2 a couple of comfortable chairs;
3 a number of straight-backed chairs;
4 two or three soft bean bags;
5 gymnastic mats;
6 a mattress;
7 a drum and tambourine;
8 a facility for playing tapes and records;
9 some method of adjusting the light in the room;
10 a video camera.

Of all these requirements I believe the most important to be space and privacy. The need for space is obvious and it is very difficult to create a mood of safety and trust for the client in a corridor or a room that necessitates constant interruption. Although I have in the past worked in very unsuitable environments I do not think it does our clients any service to 'make do' when unsuitable spaces are offered.

CASE ILLUSTRATIONS

'Susie' was a young woman of 25 years with profound learning dif-ficulties, no speech but good general physical ability. She was very isolated and withdrawn and after spending most of her life in institutional care she was now living with her mother and younger sister and attending a day centre. She was referred to me by her key worker at the day centre – 'to improve eye contact and personal interaction and to try to reduce her tedious rocking movements'. Initially I asked if I could observe Susie during her normal day at the centre and I spent a couple of hours there one morning to enable me to put her referred 'problems' into context.

I noticed that her rocking movements had a definite rhythm and meaning. When her attention was not focused she would stare vacantly into space and maintain a fairly slow, gentle, forward–backward rock. If there was any unwanted intrusion the rocking became fiercer and faster and she would avoid all eye contact with the intruder. Then, suddenly, she would laugh very loudly and run to another part of the room where she would revert to her previous rocking rhythm. Occasionally she would sit and become absorbed in drawing, making thick, clear, continuous strokes right across the paper, filling page after page, using a crayon of just one colour – black – although there were many to choose from. She became absorbed in 'washing up'. Although little attempt was made to actually clean the cups and plates, she handled them quite delicately and was intent on 'playing' with the water. She filled the cups and emptied one into another, holding a cup high and watching the water pour into the bowl. Susie avoided all physical and eye contact apart from with a couple of members of staff and one or two other day centre clients. With these particular people she would occasionally tuck her arm under one of theirs and take them for a walk around the room, laughing with glee if they were co-operative. If they would not co-operate she would pull and pull for a little while and then break off and go into her fast rocking rhythm. These observations told me a little about Susie. She was not totally autistic. She was selectively sociable. She used her rocking movements to express her boredom, frustration, or anger. She was selectively interested in her environment and could be mischievous. Considering her difficulties I decided that her coping mechanisms were not unreasonable. Remember Susie had no speech to express her antipathy to certain individuals or her desire for contact with others. She was unable to say 'No thank you, I'd rather not' when required to do something. She had found other ways, but they were not easily understood by others. That slow, vacant rocking seemed to express boredom and the faster rhythm frustration or anger. She avoided physical and eye contact where she felt little empathy but actively sought it in other cases. I did not feel that it would be appropriate to work with Susie to extinguish her coping mechanisms without something to offer in their place.

I decided not to work with Susie because of the overriding ethical consideration that it cannot be right to change an individual's behaviour simply because we do not understand it or that it is not perceived as 'normal', providing that behaviour is not harmful to others or to the individual themselves.

I discussed my observations with Susie's key worker and explained my reasons for rejecting the referral, highlighting how privileged I was to have had the opportunity for a 'bird's eye view' without personal interaction, since few of the staff actually working with Susie had such opportunities. Her key worker decided to discuss my observations with the other members of the staff and inform me of any decisions they might reach.

Four weeks later I received a report from the day centre stating that following my visit the staff had decided on a programme for Susie involving a more positive response to her behaviour. Her fierce rocking movements had reduced considerably and the staff considered that up to that stage the programme had been so successful that a return visit was requested for similar movement observations with other day centre clients. The report stated that a different perspective would be a valued development to their work.

I did return to the day centre many times and ultimately many of their clients came to me for DMT which work was followed up by day centre staff in their implementation of clients' individual development programmes.

John

John was a boy of 20 years with cerebal palsy and mild learning difficulties. His speech was very garbled and difficult to understand. His arms and legs were atrophied and spastic. He could not walk. He could understand and co-operate well and he had a very sunny disposition.

I had been seeing John once a week for about six weeks. We had been doing a lot of floor work, lots of contact, body moulding, and slow, fluid movements to ease his frequent muscle spasms. We had a good rapport. On one particular morning John arrived for his session in his wheelchair looking unusually glum. When I prepared to get him out of his chair he quite clearly said 'No!' and squirmed and wriggled and frowned. Eventually, after great communication difficulty, I understood that he wanted to stay in his chair and stretch his arms up above his head. I knew, from discussions with the physiotherapist, that this was John's greatest difficulty. He could get his arms to shoulder height and then the muscles would go into strong and painful spasm. I knew this was going to be a challenge. I suggested to John that he should forget about his arms and try to keep them still and peaceful on the arms of his wheelchair. I found a tape of some gentle Mozart and we sat peacefully listening to the music for a little while. Then I said, 'John, I want you to think for a moment and try to imagine a beautiful star, hovering, just a little way in front of you.' John gave a smile and the music continued gently in the background. I said, 'John, watch that star as it hovers. It is so light and beautiful, and it is beginning to rise higher and higher.' Very slowly, John's head moved until he was looking right up at the ceiling, but his arms were still on the chair and quite relaxed. I turned the music down slowly until it was very soft and said, 'John, the star is drifting far away until we can no longer see it. You can look at me now.' I stopped the music and he was looking at me and smiling. I told him that we had come to the end of the session and that I would see him the following week. He was furious and shouted at me, he wanted to carry on. He left gesticulating wildly. I could not understand but I am sure that he called me a few colourful names. The following week John arrived looking a bit fierce and also a little questioning. I suggested that we should repeat the previous week's session and he was very enthusiastic. So we repeated the session exactly the same: same music, same words, and same reactions from John. I said, 'I think we'll do it just once more and then we can go on to other things.' When we got to the point where the star was above his head, I gently increased the volume of the music and I said, 'Now you can really see that star John. It is not very far away. Very slowly and gently reach up and touch it. Slowly–slowly–slowly.' There he was! Head back, arms stretching up to the ceiling, no spasms, just pure joy! I will never forget the expression on John's face when he found himself reaching up without pain. If there was one single moment which convinced me that this work was worthwhile then I think that was it. Such a small thing to do – lift one's arms high in the air – but this is the 'window into feelings' that I mentioned earlier. I continued to work with John and we had many more joyful moments. He was eventually transferred to a hostel closer to his home and I lost contact with him.

Jane

Jane was a young woman of 19 years with a mild learning difficulty. She was very loud, hyperkinetic, and rather ungainly and clumsy. She was generally of a happy disposition but could be sulky at times.

I worked with Jane in a mixed group of six similar young adults, all with mild learning difficulties. My attention was focused on Jane because within the group she was very disruptive and attention seeking. I requested that she be withdrawn from the group for individual sessions.

Jane's perception of herself was of being rather fat and heavy and consequently she had adjusted her posture and gait to accommodate that perception. She always wore jeans and big, floppy sweaters or tee-shirts. In fact she was tall, slim, nicely proportioned and had no physical disability.

I was working in a fairly large studio with floor to ceiling mirrors along one wall. We began our first session by warming up the body. Rubbing arms, legs, feet, hands, backs, faces, etc., and then really shaking them out to release any tension. I asked Jane to accompany me to the back of the studio and walk down with me towards the mirrors, really looking at herself all the time. She found it very difficult to look at herself and the closer to the mirror we got the more difficult this became. Jane looked everywhere but at herself. I suggested that we try again. This time I would look at her in the mirror and she could watch me. This she managed fairly well with a lot of giggling and poking me in the ribs. I decided to stop the mirror work for a while. I reminded Jane that it was difficult to move freely wearing tight jeans and told her that she was welcome to change into leotard and tights of which I had a reasonable collection from which she could choose. Initially she was a little reticent but she did finally choose a pair of black, footless tights and a bright red leotard, and off she went to change. She returned very self-consciously and I immediately told her that she looked wonderful. 'Let's walk down to the mirror again!' I said. This time Jane managed one or two quick glimpses of herself but she maintained her ungainly gait and made many shrinking and body-covering movements.

Over a period of six months with weekly, hour-long DMT sessions, much work was directed towards Jane's body awareness and integration of the physical and inner states. Working together, facing the mirror, we identified body parts and discovered their range of movement. Moving the whole body in the immediate space – in front of *me*, behind *me*, beside *me*, etc. Stretching vertically and horizontally. Awareness of the body in motion through the whole space – walking high on the balls of the feet, running using the whole foot, crawling, rolling. Initiating and remembering pathways and spatial patterns. All of this work repeated without the mirror. Some of the work repeated with the eyes closed to emphasize the inner feeling. During this time Jane gained the ability to create her own short dance sequences and displayed obvious enthusiasm and confidence. She began to wear more attractive clothes – blouses, skirts, and pretty shoes. Her posture and gait became more synchronous with her physique although she was still occasionally clumsy in some of her movements.

After almost seven months of individual work I invited Jane to rejoin the original group.

Jane did rejoin the group and integrated herself with little difficulty. She was no longer disruptive and became a valued and creative member of the group.

I worked with this group for almost two years as part of a further education programme. They all successfully went on to sheltered work situations. Jane went to work at a local riding school.

CONCLUSIONS

I have chosen the previous case illustrations to highlight one or two particular points. Dance and movement are powerful vehicles for change. People with learning difficulties sometimes develop bizarre movement behaviours as coping mechanisms for inner states and physical tensions which, unless they can be positively replaced with more acceptable behaviour, should perhaps be left intact, the guiding principle being whether these behaviours are harmful or harming.

Dance movement therapy is particularly appropriate for people with profound physical disability as it operates psychologically as well as physically. In 'John's' case it was necessary to motivate him to utilize one of the primitive reflex patterns available to him to help him achieve his goal. This particular reflex, the symmetrical tonic neck reflex, originates in the neck muscles and is brought into play by raising or lowering the head. Raising the head results in increased extension of the arms. The tonic reflexes are most obvious during normal development, but, as previously mentioned, they are seen to dominate muscle tone in brain-damaged children or adults. Knowledge of these tonic reflexes helps us to identify their influence on posture and movement and provides starting points for therapy.

As we saw in 'Jane's' case, the acquisition of a realistic and positive body image is important to the whole psychomotor development of the individual. At the earliest stages of development it is through the body and our perception of it that we experience the world. Body image forms an essential part in the relationship between the ego and the environment. A poor or confused body image can lead to further disorders especially *motor* – clumsiness, poor co-ordination, lack of control of postural and balance mechanisms. The therapist needs to develop strategies and techniques suitable to the needs of individual clients.

SUMMARY

'If I could tell you what I mean, I would not have to dance it' was a remark attributed to Isadora Duncan. Dance is non-verbal expression and as such is difficult to describe adequately in writing. I hope, however, that I have introduced in this chapter some of the basic theory underlying DMT with this population and demonstrated its value as a tool to restore harmony where it is lacking and effect change where it is beneficial.

We have had a cursory look at one or two techniques which may be be usefully developed with personal insight and experience.

The case illustrations were chosen to elucidate theories I consider to be especially important with these clients but, as I set out to interest and enthuse, I have had to be selective so as not to overwhelm with too great a range of clinical material and detail.

The trained therapist should be confident, trustworthy, and trusting. Trust the dance, inquire for meaning, and the steps will follow.

REFERENCES

Ayres, A.J. (1975) *Sensory Integration and Learning Disorders*, Los Angeles, CA: Western Psychological Services.
Bender, L. and Boas, F. (1941) 'Creative dance in therapy', *American Journal of Psychiatry* 2: 235–44.
Feldenkrais, M. (1966) *Body and Mature Behaviour*, New York: International Universities Press.

King, L.J. (1974) 'A sensory integrative approach to schizophrenia', *American Journal of Occupational Therapy* October.

Sutherland, J. (1980) 'The British object-relations theorists: Balint, Winnicott, Fairbairn, Guntrip', *Journal of the American Psychoanalytic Association* 28: 4.

Winnicott, D. (1971) *Playing and Reality*, New York: Penguin.

BIBLIOGRAPHY

Bulowa, M. (1979) *Before Speech: The Beginning of Interpersonal Communication,* Cambridge: Cambridge University Press.

Claxton, G. (1980) *Cognitive Psychology, New Directions*, London: Routledge & Kegan Paul.

Klein, M. (1975) *Writings of Melanie Klein*, Vols 1–3, London: Hogarth.

Maher, M. and McDevitt, J. (1982) 'Thoughts on the emergence of the self with particular emphasis on the body self', *Journal of the American Psychoanalytic Association* 30: 4.

McGrew, W.C. (1972) *An Ethological Study of Children's Behaviour*, London: Academic Press.

Wells, K. (1971) *Kinesiology*, Eastbourne, Sussex: W. B. Saunders.

Chapter 11

The Action Profile® system of movement assessment for self development

Pamela Ramsden

INTRODUCTION

The Action Profile® system of assessment is based on a specific type of detailed movement observation and is a method for enabling individuals to understand their natural way of thinking things through and turning that thinking into action. It helps a person to be more aware of his or her unique style of solving problems, making decisions, and taking action. The natural energy that a person is born with and which develops as he or she matures is a potential for success and fulfilment which can be enhanced through awareness of the 'Action Profile' pattern.

The profile is currently used primarily as a tool for management development. It helps companies to position managers in the most appropriate jobs to bring out the natural potential and to develop new skills in the best possible way. The aim of this chapter is to give the reader an understanding of what Action Profile assessment is and how it can be used for self development.

The aim of the profile is not to change or 'fix' people, but rather to draw out more fully the capacity already within each person. The purpose is to create the possibility of self-fulfilment by enabling people to act in accordance with deep-seated motivations. As a result, individuals are able to think and act more effectively, manage the decision-making process, and secure the commitment of members of a team or group.

The Action Profile pattern reveals core motivational forces in the personality; therefore, an awareness of it can provide an anchor for one's development in attitude and behaviour. These core motivational forces are all called Action Motivation. The profile simply represents distributions of Action Motivation; therefore, they are not good or bad and there are no good or bad profiles. It follows that there is little value in trying to change the profile itself. Instead, any change should be geared toward altering conditions, attitudes, or assumptions that stand in the way of one's full potential of Action Motivation being completely expressed.

The Action Profile assessment is based upon a simple model of decision-making initiative and includes:

1 the process and staging of decision-making;
2 interaction during that process;
3 the overall intensity or level of the decision-making energy (dynamism);
4 adaptability in decision-making;
5 the level of identification with the environment and initiatives of others.

The assessment of an Action Profile system is based upon highly detailed observation of minute variations of movement. This gives the system its objectivity, its accuracy, and its capacity to identify deep-seated motivational forces in the personality.

Validation and reliability research has been steadily pursued along a number of avenues. A high level of inter-judge reliability between qualified Action Profile practitioners has been achieved and is systematically maintained through Action Profilers International. A valuable and comprehensive programme of validation research has been carried out by Professor Deborah Du Nann Winter over the last seven years (Du Nann Winter 1987).

The Action Profile system has a long history beginning with the brilliant work of Rudolf von Laban (Laban and Lawrence 1947) with his extraordinary insights into the nature of human movement and his development of methods for recording it. He was followed by the original pioneering work of Warren Lamb (Lamb 1965) who made the outstanding discovery of *Posture–Gesture Merging* in movement and its relationship to authenticity in behaviour. He added the dimension of *Shaping* the activity task to Laban's original concept of making the *Effort* to complete the activity, and the concepts of *Assertion* and *Perspective*. He established the original method of analysis and developed the framework of decision-making after fifteen years of painstaking research into the characteristics of different managerial functions and the decision-making process in action. He was the first to develop the *Top Team Planning* approach to top management effectiveness.

My crystallization of the theory of Action Motivation, placing it in the context of theories of motivation, helped bring the profile to its present state. There is now a clearer framework, an expansion of the Framework of Interaction and Overall Factors, a refinement of measurement of the profile and methods for teaching the system.

Theory

Action Motivation is a deep-seated drive to make decisions and take action according to an individual pattern of preferences. It could be described as the drive to express one's individuality in 'action', as it integrates two functions: (1) what would normally be seen as purely cognitive or mental functioning and (2) the physical aspects of taking initiative and putting it into practice.

An important step towards mastering the mental and physical aspects of a particular task is to achieve 'thought in action'. Action thinking could be seen as useful intelligence. It is the capacity to take the higher functions of the mind, such as imagination, conceptualization, memory, visualization, logic, etc., and perform them as an integral part of decision-making and taking action.

We all know the difference between a theoretical decision which remains 'a nice thing I might like to do one day' and a real decision which carries a commitment and inner compulsion to put it into action. A theoretical decision remains in the head, made by the mind only; a real decision reaches the body as well. The urge to get on with it is felt as much physically as it is mentally. A real decision integrates the body and the mind.

Another important impulse of the motivation comes from the integration of two aspects of the personality which also combine body and mind. These are: (a) the learning, coping, changing, executive, 'doing' part of the personality and termed 'gestural personality'; (b) the maintaining, sustaining, holding, 'being' part of the personality or the 'postural personality'.

a) Gestural personality

The first can be termed the 'gestural' personality because it enables us to use parts of ourselves singly or in combination in order to experiment, try out, venture, engage, or disengage. Technical perfection of any activity will come from the honing of the physical and mental 'gestures' or personality parts that are required in the activity, and combining them into a fluent, well co-ordinated pattern. The 'gestural personality' is expressed physically as gestures, that is, movements of isolated parts of the body, singly or in combination.

b) Postural personality

The second aspect could be termed the 'postural' personality because it enables us to 'take on' different roles, attitudes, and ways of being. It enables us to hold on to and stabilize required or desired 'personas' or ways of being. It enables us to 'be' authoritative, friendly, shy, aggressive, fatherly, motherly, nonchalant, timid, etc. It enables us to take on an appropriate attitude which, in turn, sets us up in the right way to perform a certain task or take certain types of action. The 'postural personality' is expressed physically by postural movements, that is, movements which involve the whole body in a unified expression.

As a result of the integration of gestural and postural personality there is a particular mastery. The integration of these two aspects of the personality provides a state of mind and body in which the flexible, trying out, 'doing' characteristics are backed up by an appropriate and supportive attitude or way of 'being'. This means the individual has a high degree of personal investment in the resulting behaviour. The person is not just 'trying out' a particular action or skill, not 'trying on' a particular role or attitude but has 'become' the action. The 'being' and 'doing' aspects of the personality have been combined. The person 'does' what they 'are' and 'is' what they 'do'.

The combination of these two aspects of the personality is what distinguishes true mastery of a particular task, function, skill, or art from mere technical competence. It is what makes the difference between a truly great or peak performance, and one that demonstrates technical expertize and intensity but lacks the mysterious ingredient to turn it into a memorable individual masterpiece.

When a person is able to sustain peak performance, they attain a high level of technical competence over the various parts of the chosen activity. They also develop an appropriate attitude that enables total commitment to the activity. They then bring the two together, which requires the capacity to turn a mechanical, if highly competent performance of various skills into a unified individualized expression of the individual's talent. No other person could perform the same task or activity in quite the same way.

This same process occurs whenever we learn a new skill to the point where it is no longer an extra bit grafted onto us but has become an integral part of the way we behave, or, indeed, 'who we are'. Because of this, no two persons with the same level of technical competence will perform an activity or task with precisely the same effect.

At the root of this ability is our capacity to integrate the 'gestural' and 'postural' aspects of the personality, that is, to 'become' what we 'do'. Physically this is expressed through the merging of postural movement (whole body unified) and gestural movement (isolated part of the body), i.e. 'Posture Gesture Merging' (PGM) or 'Integrated Movement'.

When the gestural and the postural personalities combine, they become the driving force of Action Motivation. Action Motivation has two compelling components: (a) the will to pursue a particular activity based upon the integration of body and mind. This leads to 'action thinking' which requires the whole body and the whole person and results in committed decision-making and action. (b) The satisfaction gained from performing the activity purely for its own sake regardless of any end result. This derives from the fulfilment of 'being' what we 'do' and finding a way of performing a task that is uniquely ours.

Motivation from within

Action Motivation is simply a drive to deal with and act on the environment in a way that is consistent with one's own natural source of energy. Acting in a way that is in tune with one's inbuilt energy preferences is satisfying in itself: the reward is self-acceptance.

This does not mean self-congratulation or complacency. It means recognition that there is a uniquely fashioned core of energy within each individual which is just that – energy, neither good nor bad in itself, just whatever it is. Self-acceptance of this nature is one of the most fulfilling, positive, and life-enhancing states for human beings to achieve.

The individual movement pattern

For every individual, the complex and unceasing interplay of movement qualities forms a pattern which is one of the most telling expressions of a person's individuality. Movement pattern is as unique and characteristic as fingerprints, while the beginning and end positions a person takes are learned habits and skills. While positions are reflective of race, class, or social upbringing, movement quality is indicative of individual motivation (Bartenieff and Lewis 1980).

There is a difference between the way in which a natural movement quality is performed and the way in which an acquired or learned movement quality is performed.

There are some important distinctions to be made, because even movement qualities can be adopted by people with an aptitude for such learning. Most proficient actors are particularly good at it. However, learned movement qualities that do not appear in the natural pattern can only be performed (a) by an isolated part of the body or (b) by the whole body 'en bloc' in a single unified expression. The first is called *Gestural* movement and the second *Postural* movement. As mentioned above there is a third possibility which is *Posture–Gesture Merging (PGM)* (Lamb and Watson 1979) or *Integrated* movement. PGM or integrated movement happens when a movement quality, say *accelerating*, begins in a *gesture* (a movement of an isolated part of the body such as the head). The accelerating continues in the *gesture* but at the same time travels into the rest of the body, becoming a whole body movement known as *posture* movement. Alternatively, PGM can take place when a particular movement quality such as accelerating is expressed first in a unified whole body movement (posture) and then flows without interruption into one body part such as a foot gesture.

When there is continuity between the gestural and the postural movement, the observer senses the consistency. When someone politely presents a hand to shake yours, you sense the use of body parts: gestural movement. When someone genuinely is interested to make your acquaintance, he or she she reaches out with the hand and the whole body follows: PGM. Because one movement flows from a single part into the whole body, PGMs are considered 'Integrated' movements. The movement statement is unified. Integrated movement is always completely individual. A person playing a series of instruments simultaneously (a literal one-man-band) is performing a gesture system, not a posture–gesture merging. If, however, they stood to take up the trumpet, they might claim a stance for their performance. Unifying the body in one movement, they might take on a 'hey, listen to me' attitude. This is a postural movement. If they returned to be seated at the drum, and if they took their feet off the foot pedals and just concentrated on the brushing, allowing the movement from their hands to flow into the whole body and back into the hands again you would see a PGM taking place, and it would be performed according to movement qualities present within their natural movement pattern.

The distinction between gesture, posture, and PGM is important because we are concerned to isolate the movement qualities that are part of the natural pattern of action motivation and not acquired attitudes or learned skills. Hence, 'it is only Posture–Gesture Merging movement that is used as a basis for analysis and construction of the Action Profile' pattern pattern (Ramsden 1973: 89).

The psychological significance of PGM has been theorized by Dr Judith Kestenberg (Kestenberg 1975). Using Freud's model of personality structure, gestures represent the ego, the part of the self which is active in and copes with the world. Postures represent the superego, the part which judges, approves, disapproves, and acts as the conscience for the ego. When gesture integrates with posture the ego is acting with approval from the superego. The psyche is in harmony.

Further research[1] has revealed that gestures are flexible, adaptable, highly functional, and are used to cope in the most efficient way with our social and physical environment. Postures portray attitudes or states of mind. They put us in the right frame of mind for a particular job and are less easy to change. Hence the integration of posture and gesture denotes the integration of the effective capacity to act in combination with the appropriate attitude or mental state.

Movement quality

To obtain the many rich and varied qualities of movement that we do, we vary the intensity and combination of what are known as movement elements. Most people do not notice their own movement variations, but are intuitively sensitive to these changes in others.

Movements elements fall into two different categories: *Effort* and *Shaping*. There follows an overview of these categories.

Effort

In terms of the effort (or assertion) quality of a movement we can vary the focus, the pressure, the timing, and the degree of control or kind of flow with which it is done. Each of these elements of variation can be considered a continuum, with a neutral area between each extreme. The four effort elements with their polarities (extremes) are as shown in Figure 11.1.

FOCUS

| Indirecting (diffuse focus) | Neutral | Directing (pinpoint focus) |

PRESSURE

| Decreasing pressure (light) | Neutral | Increasing pressure (strong) |

TIME

| Decelerating | Neutral | Accelerating |

FLOW

| Freeing (Decrease control) | | Binding (Increase control) |

Figure 11.1 The four effort elements with their polarities

Shaping

We can vary the process of shaping a movement in the following ways, based on a three-dimensional division of space: horizontal (side/side), vertical (up/down), sagittal (back/front) plane, or according to an overall taking up of space (i.e., the body can literally take up more or less space). The bodily shaping referred to here is two-dimensional sculpting of space. In horizontal or table plane shaping for instance the body curves either forward and outwards or backward and inwards to give a round gathering and scattering or enclosing and spreading-type movement.

In vertical or door plane shaping the body curves either sideways and upward or sideways and downward to give a rounded ascending (or descending) movement. In sagittal or wheel plane shaping the body curves either vertically and forward or vertically and backward to give a curving, bulging, or hollowing, advancing or retreating movement. The four dimensions of shaping are shown in Figure 11.2.

	Horizontal Plane (Table)	
Spreading	Neutral	Enclosing
	Vertical Plane (Door)	
Ascending	Neutral	Descending
	Sagittal Plane (Wheel)	
Advancing	Neutral	Retreating

Figure 11.2 Four dimensions of shaping

The variation along any of the dimensions, either of effort or shaping, can occur to any degree and in any combination with the other elements.

Movement and motivation

When a particular movement quality is experienced in a movement which integrates posture and gesture it triggers an associated conscious thought process. Because, by its very nature, a particular movement quality enables a particular type of action, it requires the conscious brain to match it with a particular type of thinking.

Directing movement for instance enables focused action, so it requires the brain to provide focused thinking. The movement quality is so perfectly what it is that it must be accompanied by the appropriate thought process.

For example to move in an integrated directing way and at the same time to be thinking in a wandering, unfocused fashion is a contradiction in terms and probably impossible to do. Such a contradiction can only be expressed by splitting the body up into contradicting gesture system or posture/gesture systems. It is questionable whether consistent **action thinking** of any type can be performed while the body is splintered into different movement qualities.

Each polarity of each movement quality engenders two associated thought processes. Each pair of thought processes has a particular outcome, for example, when a person does a *directing* movement, they are able to focus energy toward one point. When it is done with an integration of posture and gesture and the person 'becomes' what he is 'doing', all of his attention can be channelled towards a specific point.

This pinpoint focusing of attention enables the person to probe for information and to make distinctions between one thing and another. Probing for information reveals more and more specific items of data. Making distinctions gives greater and greater definition to the information by revealing how one piece is different from another. As a result of this the person is able to make a precise analysis of a situation.

Figure 11.3 shows, in diagram form, a detail of each of the action motivations which links with how they relate to movement qualities, mental processes, and outcome.

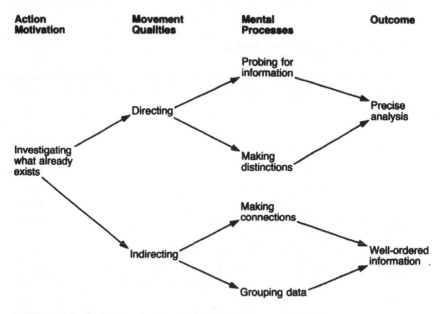

Figure 11.3 Attending to the potential for action (investigating)

When a person does *indirecting* movements (see Figure 11.3) they are able to focus energy in a way that connects several different points. When it is done with PGM it means that all the attention is channelled in a way that connects one focus of attention with another. As result the person is able to make connections between one facet of the information and another. It enables them to see which aspects are similar to each other. This in turn enables them to group items of information together under different headings and classifications. As a result they are able to put the information in order so it can be easily understood.

When *enclosing* PGM movements (see Figure 11.4) are done, the individual is able to move through and embrace a variety of different vantage points in relation to the surrounding environment.

This enables possibilities to be brought together from a number of different angles. This in turn enables toleration of apparently opposing ideas within the same sweep of attention and hence the encompassing of diverse possibilities within the scope of interest. The result is varied ways of approaching a situation.

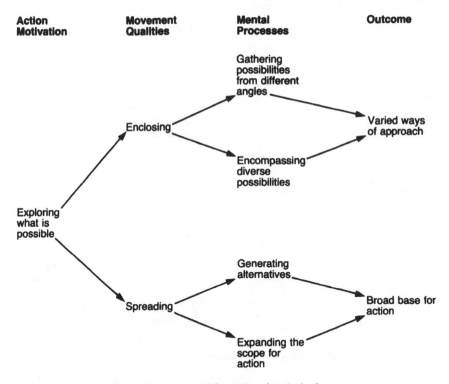

| Action Motivation | Movement Qualities | Mental Processes | Outcome |

Figure 11.4 Attending to the potential for action (exploring)

Spreading PGM movements (see Figure 11.4) allow a person to open up to and scan an increasingly broad view of the surroundings. This means that a number of different ways to approach a situation can be seen and that alternative options can be generated. It means also that it can be seen that the scope for action can be expanded and more is possible than was originally appreciated. This creates a broad base for action.

With *increasing pressure* or firm PGM movements (see Figure 11.5) a person is able to put all their body weight behind actions. By applying this firm, weighty energy to what is needed all the reasons and feelings in favour or against a particular intention can be stacked up with a sense of firmness which fuels the strength of their resolve. When events or opposition occur which might detract from this resolve even more pressure can be applied and adverse pressure resisted in order to sustain their case. This leads to the formation of a strong base for action which will not be dispelled by counter-arguments or influences.

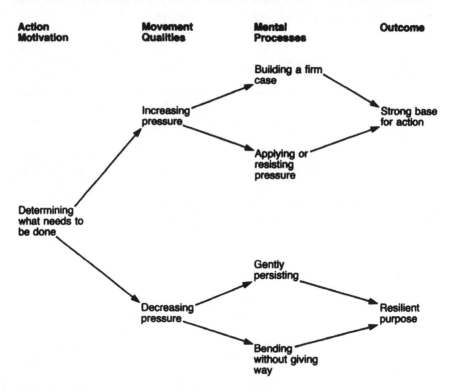

Figure 11.5 Intending to take action (determining)

When *decreasing pressure* or 'light' PGM movements are used (see Figure 11.5), the person is able to literally 'float' above a situation. It requires strength to be light for the weight of the body must be rarefied in order to create the sensation of overcoming gravity. This means that the person has the strength gently to persist with their intention. When obstacles arise, or when thoughts or arguments are brought to bear which could undermine them, they simply bend with the force of the blow, but then spring back again. There is no giving way. Thus the purpose is resiliently pursued.

Descending movements (see Figure 11.6) enable a person to get beside and below whatever they are facing. This means they can gain a sense of proportion about how big or small whatever is in front of them is in relation to themselves. This type of perspective enables them to judge the relative importance of various events and factors and establish whether there are issues which they should take into consideration. In any situation they are able to assess the relevant issues. By continuing to assess the relative 'size' or importance of various issues they are able to say which is the most important, which the second most important, and so on, that is, they are able to rank the issues in order of importance. Knowing the relative importance of whatever they are facing enables them to establish realistic priorities.

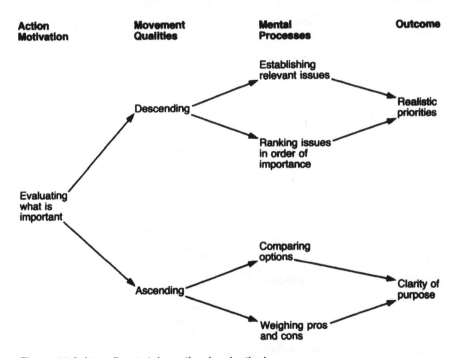

Figure 11.6 Intending to take action (evaluating)

When, on the other hand, a person does *ascending* PGM movements they move beside and above whatever they are facing. This provides a way of looking down on and comparing one thing with another in terms of their size in relation to each other and to themselves. This means they can become clear about the nature of their relevance. In addition they can compare different aspects of the same options or factors. Thus they can weigh pros and cons in relation to what they now know are the most relevant criteria. This will crystallize why they think a particular option or factor is more important. Because they now know not only what is important but also why it is important they are able to be clear about their purpose.

With an *accelerating* PGM movement (see Figure 11.7) a person can do just that – accelerate or speed up both physically and mentally. Accelerating should not be confused with 'fast'. Accelerating requires a change of pace: from one pace to a faster pace. It means that a person is able to speed up the pace of their activity and to seize opportunities. To seize an opportunity one needs to be in a state of alert readiness. This attitude to time and the passing of events predisposes a person to notice opportunities and enables them to speed up enough to seize them before the moment passes. This provides a facility for opportune action.

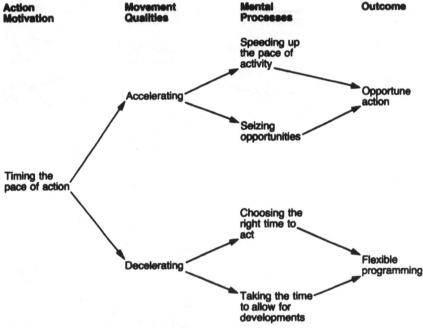

Figure 11.7 Committing to action (timing)

Decelerating PGM involves the physical process of slowing down, which in turn promotes a calm attitude of mind in which it is possible to perceive that the right amount of time for any desired action is available. The person feels able to stretch time out and thereby slow events down. There is no rush, hence the person can calmly choose the right moment to act. They can take the time to allow for certain events or developments to take place of their own accord, thus maximizing the appropriateness of whatever actions they initiate. As a result the person can programme their interventions in a flexible way in tune with the changing pace of other events.

When a person does *retreating* PGM (see Figure 11.8) they are able to distance themselves from whatever they are aiming for. They are in a better position to see what steps and stages they will need to go through in order to attain a particular goal. Hence they can plan the stages before taking any action. As they progressively assess what stages are needed, what stages have been accomplished and what is still left to do, they are able to measure their progress. This means that they create step-by-step action plans which are constantly kept alive and up-to-date according to the latest progress.

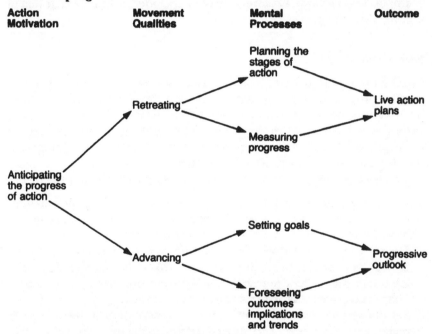

| Action Motivation | Movement Qualities | Mental Processes | Outcome |

Figure 11.8 Committing to action (anticipating)

The movement of *advancing* PGM enables a person to see further ahead and to get closer to whatever is ahead of them. This enables them to mentally transport themselves towards a desired place in the future. As a result they can set goals for themselves. By constantly looking ahead they can foresee what the outcome of a particular train of events will be, the current trends and the implications of a particular course of action. This results in a forward-looking and progressive outlook.

TECHNIQUES

The Action Profile pattern is drawn up by observing the client's integrated (PGM) movement during an interview. The movement preferences are resolved and expressed as percentages. By understanding their own and others' preferences in these terms managers can avoid unnecessary misunderstandings and conflict and can even deliberately call on each other's complementary strengths. A manager who is low in *investigating* for instance, instead of being frustrated by those who like probing and detailed work, can deliberately call on such people to provide well-analysed information that otherwise would be lacking. Profiles are used to examine the balance of motivation within operating teams. Sometimes teams are even put together bearing the profiles of members in mind so as to create a particular emphasis. For example, several high 'explorers' may be included to ensure that lots of possibilities are generated.

Self development

Profiles are also used to improve the personal effectiveness of individuals and to provide a basis for significant self development. Individuals need opportunities to realize their potential and ultimately become managers of their own motivations, skills, and capacities. Awareness of deep-seated motivations can serve as an anchor for the integrated development of new skills and behaviours.

Self development is conducted according to the following principles:

1 Recognize that the Action Profile pattern is simply energy – neither good nor bad in itself. It only becomes appropriate or inappropriate depending on how it is expressed in a given situation.
2 Recognize that individuals need to conform to their action motivation as fully as possible. In so doing they are able to have a high degree of job satisfaction. Their motivation is high and they are more effective. They take more initiative and can be more creative.
3 For maximum personal effectiveness it is necessary to learn how to orchestrate your own and others' action motivations in relation to the demands of the various tasks, roles, and situations you have to manage. In order to do this the following areas of knowledge and skills are required.
    a) You need to know what motivations are truly necessary for what situations, remembering that your instinctive tendency is to feel there is more need for your own high areas than may be the case.
    b) You need to know how to rely on, develop, and exploit your high areas. The more you can gravitate towards situations that

genuinely require your high motivations in full strength, the more fulfilled and effective you will be.

c) You need to know how to hold high motivations in check when they are *not* needed and how to increase or compensate for low motivations when they *are* needed.

d) High areas can be used to compensate for low areas. Strategies can be developed that achieve the same result as the application of a certain action motivation but through a different means.

A word of caution

Any control or modification of the natural pattern needs to be done with sensitivity and care. Too severe or prolonged alteration will lead to loss of satisfaction, initiative, and ultimately one's productivity. It can also damage psychological and physical health. Sometimes it is possible to expend far too much effort in overcoming low areas of motivation. It will be damaging and self-defeating to focus all your energy on overcoming your low areas, while ignoring and taking for granted your high areas.

A person may develop a habit of focusing too much on low areas if they spend a long time in a situation where the low areas are genuinely required. Such a pattern may also develop if an individual is in prolonged contact with powerful people who are high in the areas in which he or she is low, since such people consequently put a high value on those areas. An example of this is where parents differ significantly in their Action Profile pattern from a child. A parent, for instance, who is high in *determining* will find it easy to apply discipline and persistence through pressure and force of resolve. They will tend to expect the child to achieve the same degree of discipline and persistence in the same way. The child who is low in *determining* will find this very difficult. They may be constantly punished and scolded for lack of performance, and may in turn adopt the pattern of chastising themselves and constantly 'trying' to be more determined.

CASE ILLUSTRATION

First some theoretical aspects of personality need to be mentioned as a context for the application of the Action Profile pattern in self development. It may help to view the human personality as being like an onion with many different layers (see Figure 11.9).

a) Core layers

These are fundamental, deeply entrenched energies and belief systems. We may be unaware that they underpin all our behaviour and ways of viewing the world. They are extremely difficult to change to any marked degree.

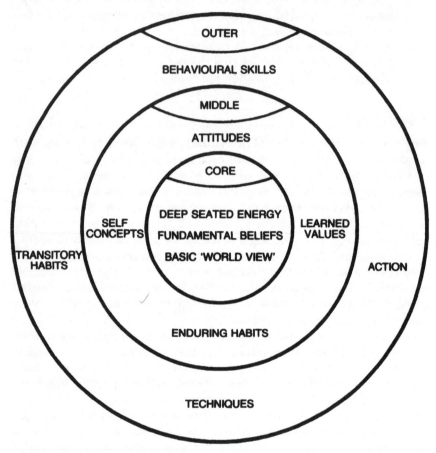

Figure 11.9 Layers of personality

b) Middle layers

These layers are likely to be attitudes and currently held beliefs and values, including perceptions of oneself as well as others, and may be negative or positive (for example, 'I am hopeless at sport'). These attitudes are based upon past experience and may or may not be relevant to the current situation.

c) Outer layers

These include behaviours which can be, with practice, readily altered and improved. They include intellectual skills, e.g., listening, questioning, and presenting, and behavioural skills, such as assertive ways of speaking and influencing others.

Dramatic personality changes will result from significant modifications at the core level. Such changes may be positive, as in a major spiritual experience, or negative, as in the case of severe nervous breakdown. Experience with the Action Profile pattern indicates that it measures core-level energies. These energies may fluctuate marginally over time, but the basic pattern does not change. A more significant change may occur during times of severe crisis or as a result of diligent effort, but in due course the individual seems to return to the original pattern.

Therefore, a change in the core energy pattern of the individual is not a sensible aim for self development work. It is far more useful to aim for increasing the competence of behaviours through which the core energies of the Action Profile pattern are expressed. The usefulness of the Action Profile pattern in self development is not in getting the profile itself to change, but in creating an awareness of the profile which enables more effective performance to take place more quickly.

Stages in development

An effective process for development is as follows:

1 Create an awareness of one's core energies through the Action Profile pattern

This gives persons a sense of stability by showing them that there is a unique pattern of motivation yielding certain basic potentials, and by providing a strong sense of self, of an identity that endures and cannot be damaged.

2 Create awareness of blockages in the middle layer

These are negative attitudes, beliefs, and self-concepts that prevent growth. Lack of confidence, for instance, will usually result from some kind of negative message 'stuck' in the brain, repeated over and over without the person being fully aware of it.

3 Establish new behavioural skills and techniques

These will enable persons to express their unique pattern of potential more competently and more in tune with the demands of their lives and professions.

These 3 stages need to be seen as a cycle where each can affect the others (see Figure 11.10).

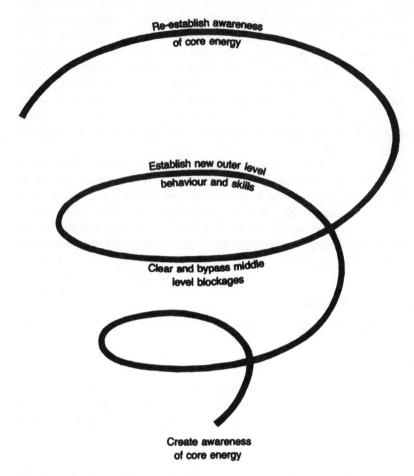

Figure 11.10 Stages in development

The need for integrated development

There are dangers from too much concentration on middle-layer development. When someone becomes overly introspective, they may lose contact with their own core characteristics. While working on changing negative attitudes and self-concepts, individuals can be manipulated by charismatic teachers to conform with extreme values and behaviours.

The safest and most effective development comes when a strong awareness of one's core characteristics provides a sense of enduring identity, which gives a stable base for development. Clear development objectives can be provided by defining what areas of performance need improvement. Intellectual and behavioural skills or techniques can be outlined to fulfil the objectives. Appropriate exercises in awareness and skill development can be developed and practised, for example, assertiveness, presentation, or negotiating skills. If difficulties and blockages appear, then work can be done to bypass negative or unhelpful attitudes and self-concepts.

Mark

Quantum leaps in self development can be achieved by working on all three levels of personality. An example of this type of development occurred with Mark, the marketing director of a large multinational company. Mark is a highly intelligent, creative, powerful individual. He has a first-rate academic track record and is highly regarded by his company. He was marketing director of one of the group's major companies when he began this development programme. Subsequently, and within a very short period of time, he went on to become managing director of the same company. This is the story of the self development of an already successful manager with enormous potential. The process described below took place over a period of approximately twelve months.

a) Core layer

The Action Profile pattern provided an anchor in this layer. Mark found the profile to be awakening and legitimizing. This applied particularly to very high areas in the profile which had previously led to behaviour Mark had tried to suppress. It was validating to realize that there was a deep-seated pattern of motivation that could not and should not be changed. Instead of suppressing his energies, it would be far more constructive to find ways of enabling his pattern to fit the needs of the situation.

b) Middle layer

For most adults, a lifetime of trying to be successful and acceptable according to the prescribed expectations of parents, teachers, and organizations leads to habits and attitudes that block and inhibit potential. The attempt to fit one's unique pattern of energies into the uniform moulds required by society usually results in some degree of distortion. It is this distortion that prevents one's true potential from being realized.

It is usually difficult, in the normal course of events, for people to change these subtle sabotaging mechanisms since they work slightly outside one's awareness. They have to be brought into consciousness, therefore, before they can be bypassed.

Many techniques for bringing blocking mechanisms into awareness are available, for example, with Mark techniques were used from Transactional Analysis such as script analysis and from Gestalt therapy such as 'Top Dog/Under Dog' conversations (James and Jongeward 1971). Techniques are also available for overlaying them with positive, constructive ideas, attitudes, and self-expectations.

In Mark's case, there was a cleverly designed set of mutually reinforcing blocking mechanisms. From childhood experiences, he carried the messages that a) he had to be always first, b) he had to be perfect, c) he would never be good enough, messages which have failure built in to them.

As most of us do, he strove valiantly and almost unceasingly (except for a short rebellious phase at about age 16) to fulfil these self-imposed instructions, and there were positive results from the instructions. Since Mark set extremely high standards for himself, he did always come first academically. He worked extremely hard to perform well at work, and he succeeded. To obey these 'instructions', Mark had somehow to force the natural and powerful motivating forces that stemmed from his core energy (Action Profile pattern) into compliance.

The key features of his profile were:

* Very high *exploring*, 30 per cent of total motivation.
* High *anticipating*, 20 per cent of total motivation.
* Very low *evaluating*, 4 per cent of total motivation.
* Low *determining*, 10 per cent of total motivation.
* Low *intention* stage (*evaluating* and *determining* together only 14 per cent).

(See p. 227 for *exploring*, p. 231 for *anticipating*, p. 229 for *evaluating*, and p. 228 for *determining*.)

He was able to use many of the benefits of the profile. His high *exploring* and high *anticipating* meant, for instance, that he could consider and select from a vast number of alternatives in a very short time. This gave him an exceptional talent for quickly coming up with precisely appropriate solutions to problems.

Mark was constantly trying to inhibit the wandering nature of his *exploring*. In addition, he was constantly trying to replace the natural flexibility of low *intention* with the consistency of purpose natural to high *intenders*. The enormous strain of this meant that he often resorted to unnecessarily manipulative methods in order to achieve what he wanted; for example, he would go to elaborate lengths in order to discredit a colleague in a meeting rather than present his opposing viewpoint in a straightforward way.

He was often able to see the need for far-reaching, innovative solutions, well ahead of others (high exploring and high anticipating). Without the full belief in his own unique way of working, however, he lacked the confidence to explain his thought processes to others. As a result, he developed the habit of speaking in a way which confused his audience.

His frustration often caused him to be extremely impatient and intolerant with others. The impossibly high expectations he had of himself meant that he had equally unattainable expectations of others.

The middle-layer work lessened to some extent Mark's subconscious taskmaster's control. Exercises such as entering total states of bodily relaxation, positive visualization affirmations, and 'inner guide' meditations (Steinbrecher 1982) allowed him to superimpose a more creative and positive layer of self-expectation.

c) Outer layer

As described above, core-layer awareness (Action Profile pattern) acts as an anchor by validating the unalterable 'rightness' of a deep-seated pattern of energy. Middle-layer work, described above, enables the individual to examine the unique set of controlling mechanisms which he or she has created. Negative aspects can be bypassed and a more positive process introduced. Thus, on the outer level, new behaviours can be acquired which allow a truer expression of the underlying core pattern.

Once Mark fully understood that his way of thinking was very different from others' and that their resistance to his ideas often came from lack of understanding rather than negativity or enmity, he was able to stop confusing and bewildering people, and unleash his latent capacity to speak with devastating precision and clarity. He was able to condense a wealth of possibilities and implications into arguments of elegant and persuasive simplicity.

Because he was now so much more tolerant of his own way of working he was able to demonstrate a far greater level of tolerance for other people's different and often slower thought processes. Instead of prematurely writing people off as incompetent, he learned to observe others more objectively and hence to create an environment where a wide variety of differing levels of ability and styles could flourish.

Instead of forcing himself to maintain *intention* (against his low *intending* nature), he took advantage of the extra time he gained by not having to go through the *intention* phase. He now gives other people the time and space they need to get through the *intention* phase and uses his *exploring* to help them through it. At a meeting, he concentrates on managing the interaction so that everyone is included in the joint *intention* forming. He may even deliberately arrange 'collisions' of opinion so that all the issues are recognized. Instead of being frustrations, meetings are now ideal opportunities for creating team work.

Mark translates his greater self-acceptance and awareness of others into a straightforward formula for effectiveness. If you prevent a person from operating in accordance with the underlying pattern of energy, you simply make them ineffective. It is true that one person's way of working may actually be more financially costly than another's. A high explorer may, for instance, need more staff, which obviously costs more. But, in the end, if it means that a major project is successful, then it is worth it.

In addition, once a person's deep-seated motivation to work in a certain way is understood and accepted, the need becomes less extreme, hence less expensive. As Mark concisely summarized, 'People who are understood tend to move toward the most efficient solution'. Finally, it is possible to use high motivations to compensate for low motivations.

When individuals are functioning in their areas of high motivation they are more comfortable and confident, and hence are more free to experiment with different ways of behaviour. It is an effective strategy, therefore, to use high motivation to set the scene for concentrating on areas of low motivation.

For example, a person who is high in *determining* but low in *anticipating* can build up a strong resolve to learn and practise anticipatory techniques and invite *anticipation* from others. A person who is high in *anticipating* but low in *determining*, on the other hand, can look ahead and *anticipate* how and when he or she will need to be *determined*. They can therefore plan to pre-empt these situations or plan how to deal with them when they arrive.

CONCLUSION

The Action Profile® system of assessment has a long history, beginning as it did with the work of Rudolf von Laban who died in 1956. Its application has become quite specific to the field of management and it is used as a map for guidance. It has its fundamental principles and understanding based firmly in the world of movement. However, the movement is translated into behavioural terms before it reaches the client.

The Action Profile system is acknowledged as one of the most powerful tools for increasing the effectiveness of individual managers and teams. In an environment which is inundated with 'quick fix' methods the Action Profile system is becoming known as a process for long-term, deep-seated development which acknowledges the dignity and true individuality of human beings in the work setting.

An application for this movement profile suitable for more general participation, one which does work directly with movement, has been developed by myself and Ellen Goldman in New York. The aim of this work is to assist participants to identify their preferred patterns of movement, to become aware of their unique integrated movement and to use this awareness for personal growth and development.[2]

NOTES

This chapter is based upon the book *Tapping Management Potential* by Pamela Ramsden and Jody Zacharias (1991), Aldershot: Gower. The phrase 'Action Profile' is a registered name.

1 Goldman, E. and Ramsden, P., unpublished research, 1988. Apply to Pamela Ramsden through the editor for details.
2 For details of courses on Integrated Movement apply to Pamela Ramsden through the editor.

REFERENCES

Bartenieff, I. and Lewis, D. (1980) *Body Movement: Coping with the Environment*, New York: Gordon & Breach.
Du Nann Winter, D. (1987) *Movement Studies: A Journal of the Laban/Bartenieff Institute of Movement Studies, Observer Agreement Field Studies and Action Profiling Reliability*, New York: Laban/Bartenieff Institute of Movement Studies.
James, M. and Jongeward, D. (1971) *Born to win*, Reading, MA: Addison Wesley.
Kestenberg, J. (1975) *Children and Parents: Psychoanalytical Studies in Development*, New York: Jason Aronson.
Laban, R. and Lawrence, F.C. (1947) *Effort*, London: Macdonald & Evans.
Lamb, W. (1965) *Posture and Gesture*, London: Duckworth.
Lamb, W. and Watson, E. (1975) *Body Code*, London: Routledge & Kegan Paul.
Ramsden, P. (1973) *Top Team Planning*, London: Cassell.
Ramsden, P. and Zacharias, J. (1991) *Tapping Management Potential*, Aldershot: Gower.
Steinbrecher, E. (1982) *The Inner Guide Meditation*, Wellingborough: The Aquarian Press.

BIBLIOGRAPHY

Moore, C. L. and Yamamoto, K. (1988) *Beyond Words: Movement Observation and Analysis*, New York: Gordon & Breach.
Moore, C. L. (1982) *Executives in Action*, Plymouth: Macdonald and Evans.

Chapter 12

The snake sheds a skin

Themes of order and chaos in dance movement therapy

Paul Tosey

The transmutation of the life–death–rebirth cycle is exemplified by the shedding of the Snake's skin. It is the energy of wholeness, cosmic consciousness, and the ability to experience anything willingly and without resistance. It is the knowledge that all things are equal in creation and that those things which might be experienced as poison can be eaten, ingested, integrated, and transmuted if one has the proper state of mind.

(Sams and Carson 1988: 61)

INTRODUCTION

This chapter's function is to stand back and connect themes and issues across the other chapters of the book. It is deliberately a non-specialist perspective, in that it draws on no direct experience of DMT as practitioner or client; my familiarity with DMT is through knowing practitioners, and my perspective is that of someone with a professional interest in human change and development across many spheres, including the psychotherapeutic and the organizational (Tosey 1986). That perspective is based largely on the work of Gregory Bateson (1973, 1979, 1988), who challenged the orthodoxies of social science and developed an epistemology based on the unity of mind and body.

The chapter is intended to demonstrate both an empathy with DMT and enough detachment from the profession to notice things that insiders might have missed. I own to having faith in DMT's validity and aim to take a critical perspective without writing a critique; but I am unqualified and inexperienced enough in the field to make connections and ask questions without being distracted by wanting to judge the detail of the contributors' practices.

The image from which the title of this chapter is taken has a dual significance. First, DMT is itself a process of healing; it aims, broadly, at transmutation, and the snake, as in the healing symbol of the caducaeus, may represent its nature. Second, this book itself is the newly shed skin of DMT, part of DMT's own life–death–rebirth cycle; and to this there are at least three aspects. First, the snake itself is no longer there, contained within the skin, so the skin is a marker, an artefact telling of an event in time, the book as a record of DMT theory and practice. Then the snake-skin says much about the creature that has since moved on; it tells of its appearance and movement, its nature and habits. It can be compared with other creatures and understood as part of an ecological system. In this way the book is also symbolic, illustrating DMT's social functions and its relationship to other practices and philosophies. 'Dance', 'movement', and 'therapy' are metaphors as well as literal descriptions, part of a pattern that reaches through history and space. Finally, at a third level this skin is as much the 'real' snake as the inside it has expelled, separated materially by time and distance but still part of the total being. This chapter explores those levels of the text and, especially, the connections between them.

ORDER AND CHAOS

I approached the book and its delightful, daunting range of contributions as I might approach a client in my own practice, curious about the metaphors and beliefs that lie within the text and aiming to draw out underlying patterns rather than comment or summarize alone.

What began to emerge from reading the chapters – or what I began to perceive in them, for this was a deliberate search and a personal sense-making – was a recurrent set of dialectics. These consisted of themes that were or could be connected as pairs, like safety and risk, and structure and improvisation (see Table 12.1 below). People such as Ken Wilber (1979), Gregory Bateson (1973), and Charles Hampden-Turner (1981) regard the tendency to identify polarities as a simple but very significant reflection of the psyche. Wilber, for example, says;

> Notice that all spatial and directional dimensions are opposites: up vs. down, inside vs. outside, high vs. low, long vs. short. . . . And notice that all things we consider serious and important are one pole of a pair of opposites: good vs. evil, life vs. death, pleasure vs. pain, God vs. Satan, freedom vs. bondage.
>
> (Wilber 1979: 15)

Wilber makes the point that these dichotomies exist by virtue of the boundaries we create. Drawing boundaries is inevitable and essential, but typically people begin to value one pole more than the other, and then cling to the positive and reject or project the negative. Thus Hampden-Turner notes that 'we use linear yardsticks of virtue that make strength "good" and weakness "bad" and we split-off this badness from us' (1981: 168). This valuing reflects a fundamental error of epistemology; it is an outcome of perception, language, and emotion, rather than being something that necessarily exists. Wilber says:

> But since all opposites are actually aspects of one underlying reality, this is like trying to totally separate the two ends of a single rubber band. All you can do is pull harder and harder – until something violently snaps.
>
> (Wilber 1979: 27)

Starhawk points out the potential depth of significance of this process of splitting: 'Light is idealized and dark is devalued. . . . The war of dark and light is the metaphor that perpetuates racism' (1982: 21). The concern of all these writers is to develop an awareness that can reconnect, embrace, and transcend the opposites.

It is inevitable, then, that paired themes will appear in and be perceivable in these accounts of DMT theory and practice. What is interesting and instructive is both the particular set of dimensions manifested, which will reflect the distinctive nature and content of DMT, and, especially, the way these dialectics are treated; this may reveal issues of DMT's identity and development as a whole. To what extent, therefore, are themes understood as complementary faces of the same whole, belonging to the same process? And to what extent are they split as opposites, seen as polarities or dichotomies of which one element is valued over the other? Is their coexistence an irony to be enjoyed or a sign of something amiss that must be rectified, a poison that can be transformed or one which is nothing but a threat? Where is there integration and transcendence, where do 'battles become dances' (Wilber 1979: 29)?

Investigating the boundaries in DMT, as reflected in the text of this book, was therefore both fascinating and helpful. The themes in the text coalesced around a higher-order dialectic of order and chaos; not surprising in two senses, first, because this archetypal theme could be explored in any text and, second, because Helen Payne's original vision for the book was about order from chaos. Order and chaos were reflected both in the major issues discussed in the book, such as the identity and aims of DMT and its practitioners, and in the accounts of practice themselves. Table 12.1 summarizes several, not necessarily all, of those related themes.

The two sections below trace these themes and explore the relationship of the dialectics. The first concentrates on the identity of DMT – its definitions, development, and relationship to other disciplines. The theme of identity has received much direct comment in the book as well as being embedded in it, and it concerns the being and transmutation

Table 12.1

Order	Chaos
structure	improvisation
safety	risk
the known	the unknown
rhythm	absence of rhythm
meaning	ambiguity
connection	disconnection
integration	fragmentation
imitation	autonomy
similarity	difference
container	contained
synchrony	asynchrony
the verbal	the non-verbal
the literal	the metaphorical
dance	movement

of DMT. The second section draws out what seemed to be five central, linked concepts of DMT theory and practice: 'synchrony', 'containers', 'meaning', 'relationship', and 'the energy of wholeness'.

THE IDENTITY OF DMT

One purpose of this book may be to help establish identity. Not only is this an explicit concern but also there are signs of anxiety about whether DMT is recognized and taken seriously. There seems to be a serious tone to the whole book; what is missing, for example from a client's account of a problem, can be as significant as what is emphasized, and I did begin to wonder where the fun is in DMT, especially since (as Penfield points out) catharsis is essentially a movement dynamic and since play is referred to as the prototype for the therapy experience (MacDonald). Fortunately, humour does appear in some of the accounts of practice; perhaps it seemed too chaotic for the theoretical sections, where it is restricted mainly to puns on movement and dance?

Order and chaos seem to lie behind the whole issue of identity in a similar way to the example of humour: a concern to become established, recognized, and accepted gives the impression of being at odds with some aspects of DMT's character. As a result there is an uneasy, unresolved feel to much of what is said about the identity of DMT, its full potential certainly represented in the book but scattered around the text rather than being articulated confidently.

Identity is described and approached explicitly from at least three directions in the book, which reflect but do not correspond exactly to the three aspects of the text-as-snakeskin. Each category has variations, and each illuminates the issue of identity.

1 Intrinsic: with reference to evolution and archetype, as a level of experience that predates and underlies many other therapies.
2 Comparative: in relation to other therapies, arts therapies, and other movement-based approaches, and as a profession.
3 Descriptive: as an activity or process, whether literally or meta-phorically, including references to DMT's goals.

1 Intrinsic definition

This first type is represented, for example, by Payne's reference to the fundamental relationship between motion and emotion, by Noack's reference to the Muse Terpsichore, and by her reference to dance as ancient: 'dance was in the beginning the sacred language through which we communed and communicated with the vast unknown'. The primary nature of the body is reflected by Merleau-Ponty, cited by Liebowitz: 'It is through my body that I understand other people and it is through my body that I perceive things.'

This holds an ambivalence: movement is primordial, ancient, and fundamental but DMT is very young, especially in the UK. DMT is also principally a female occupation: all the main contributors to this book are women, reflecting the profile of the profession. Of the three faces of the Goddess, maiden, mother, and crone (Woolger and Woolger 1990: 344), DMT seems to have aspects of both maiden and crone but little of the mother – though motherhood has recently become part of several contributors' lives. Could DMT be seen as having the strengths and the frailties of both youth and age without the stability yet of middle life?

The relative maturity of American DMT is rejected by Payne, who asserts the distinctiveness of UK and European practice. Perhaps Stanton suggests that US and UK practices are diverging, though if Jungian approaches are indeed more common in America and the psychoanalytic usually preferred in Europe, could that be a difference of developmental phase – the Jungian naturally succeeding the psychoanalytic – rather than a divergence?

Similarly, the felt pressure to follow the other UK arts therapies methodologically and developmentally, because their formal and pro-fessional structures are already in place, seems to prompt a reluctance, even a resentment, at the thought of the ancestor bowing to the progeny. Payne acknowledges the need to develop a research tradition but is concerned not to rely on 'old paradigm' methodology simply because it is conventionally acceptable. As Stockley notes, though, the acceptance of art, music, and drama as therapies 'paved the way for dance movement therapy to get on its feet'.

Perhaps there is impatience with the need to establish an identity at all. I speculate that DMT has awareness of the lesser influence of the archetypal mother and 'male' energy in its current identity, in the sense that this book urges both maturity and order. My impression is that, ironically, there is a danger for DMT of undervaluing the maiden and the crone in itself (Stockley's chapter exemplifies the quiet strength of the age of wisdom), perhaps arising from that understandable desire to become an established profession.

2 Comparative definition

The comparative references identify DMT with, and differentiate it from, other therapies and disciplines. There is an issue of the balance between distinctiveness and relatedness, and perhaps tension about what is considered superior and inferior, linked to the above comments about US practice and the other UK arts therapies.

Although 'Dance movement therapy does not align itself with any particular psychological or psychoanalytical school' (Stanton), connections to other psychotherapeutic theories, models, and practices abound. For example, Freud, Jung, Klein, Reich, Winnicott, Bowlby, Gestalt, humanistic psychology, behaviourism, and existentialism are openly acknowledged and embraced; psychotherapeutic concepts, particularly transference and counter-transference, are frequently mentioned. Penfield refers to her work as 'parallel to any other psychotherapy'.

Differentiation includes Payne's concern to say what DMT is not: not formal dance, not teaching, not occupational therapy, and not physiotherapy. MacDonald emphasizes the focus on the expressive rather than the functional qualities of movement, and that 'DMT is not simply a physical therapy'.

Between these two, the alignment and the differentiation, is the ambiguous relationship with the other arts therapies, the immediate family of DMT. An apparent frustration is that, in the experience of the contributors, either movement is felt to be treated superficially and in theoretically invalid ways or it is commandeered as belonging to others' territory. The formal definition of DMT (Payne) tries to address this, though it is of the third, descriptive type.

3 Descriptive definition

The final type of definition includes references to DMT as an activity or process, and especially to the perceived aims or outcomes of DMT. These relate to the dialectics of order and chaos especially because at times DMT is defined as something that moves between these polarities, typically from chaos to order with issues of disorder. At other times DMT is described and practised as something integrating and transcendent.

This category of definition also captures more pointedly than the previous two the variety within the field of DMT, reflecting both the considerable differences in training and background of the contributors and the range of contexts of practice.

Some of the more concrete and behavioural aims include:

- improving functioning and control
- increasing movement repertoire
- enlarging choice
- experiencing new ways of interacting with others.

Other references are more psychotherapeutic in flavour:

- making archetypal images conscious and learning to relate to them
- moving from negative to positive aspects of the Great Mother
- integrating opposites
- integrating, not ventilating, past experiences.

These two categories probably reflect the extremes, and there is much middle ground (for example, 'strengthening the sense of body image'). What does it mean that DMT spans such a range? Does it have a coherence and an identity, or is it so diverse that it is amorphous? DMT thus seems to embody in its identity a tension between formality and order (dance) and chaos (movement) – the final dialectic in Table 12.1.

My sense is that these categories do have essential connections. For example, whilst Payne differentiates DMT from teaching, where the focus is on specific learning outcomes rather than inward processes, the more concrete focus of some practitioners suggests that DMT can, if it chooses, yield specific outcomes. There is also a consistency of movement metaphor and language in the text (space, rhythm, flow, and touch) that enables the different contributions to relate to each other. What if DMT is 'both-and', not 'either-or'?

Wilber comments on the way different psychological and religious systems appear to have different and conflicting aims. He reconciles these contradictions by suggesting that 'these different approaches are actually approaches to different levels of a person's self' (1979: 11). In effect, they are all about the healing of splits, but the splits are different, for example, 'conscious and unconscious, mind and body, or total organism and environment' (1979: 12).

This also connects with Bateson's concept of levels of learning, a hierarchy of logical types from Learning O to Learning IV (1973: 258). Learning I, for example, includes 'those items which are most commonly called "learning" in the psychological laboratory' (1973:

258), or learning on the stimulus–response model, which could include practical, behavioural outcomes of DMT. Learning II denotes 'learning to learn', which in psychotherapy, Bateson says, 'is exemplified most conspicuously by the phenomena of transference' (1973: 271). This is because Learning II is about learning across contexts: transference is literally the unconscious transfer of the way one has learned to relate to another significant person, such as a parent, to the relationship with the therapist.

Bateson's model is helpful because 'no amount of rigorous discourse of a given logical type can "explain" phenomena of a higher type' (1973: 265). In other words, a behaviourist approach that is concerned with Learning I will not recognize or accept as significant issues of level II, such as transference. This does not make the Learning I approach invalid, but it does mean its scope is limited to (or focused upon) that level. A client wanting to work on issues such as identity and lifelong patterns of relating to people would need a therapist whose theory and practice embraced at least Level II.

What seems important is that DMT has the flexibility to work at these two levels, and at more. DMT can, therefore, help in practical, behavioural ways, but this does not make it only about learning new skills. The accounts of DMT in the book seem to accentuate variety and difference, perhaps in order to discriminate between DMT and non-therapeutic approaches to movement and also to establish identity, perhaps simply because it is easier to focus on and define smaller domains of activity. The resulting irony is that some attempts to establish identity (demonstrating DMT's efficacy at the behavioural level) seem to other practitioners to threaten it (if DMT becomes perceived as only about that level), potentially setting up those two approaches as opposite poles. Bateson's framework allows for a coherence that embraces apparent contradictions in purpose without collapsing their differences.

Distinctiveness and identity

The above definitions help to capture the array of possibilities within DMT; they also draw attention to a persistent puzzle of the book. That movement and dance are special, and that DMT has significant differences from other therapies, seems clear to the contributors. Putting that elusive distinctiveness into words, however, is difficult.

The most concrete aspects are, for example, that DMT is appropriate for people who have difficulty with other media; Payne refers to the suitability of DMT for those with language and learning difficulties, precisely because it does not require verbal skills. And movement, according to Birdwhistell (1970: cited, for example, in James and

Woodsmall 1988: 10) contributes 55 per cent of what we communicate, compared with 7 per cent from the words we say, so is in theory a powerful as well as a universal medium. We all symbolize in movement, a process that constitutes the essence of DMT (Penfield); and there is a movement aspect and a movement metaphor to any experience – Liebowitz, for example, refers to the movement metaphor of death as 'falling forever'. As Stockley notes, therefore, DMT can operate on 'all the levels that human movement involves; the physical or mechanical, the communicative or expressive, and the symbolic or unconscious'. Perhaps, as MacDonald says, 'the only limitation is that of the individual therapist'.

However, the price of movement's pervasiveness and primacy is that its language, being pre-verbal, is highly ambiguous. Dance is replete with meaning, but there is no clear linkage between signifier (movement) and signified (the meaning of movement). Dance performances can have standard interpretations if there is a definite story line, but paradoxically the more that movement becomes ordered through being tied to specified, shared meanings, the more it loses its rich ambiguity and potential for meaning. Dance and movement are less codified and less codifiable than other media, which may give DMT professionals some cause for regret when writing about theory and practice, but this is the very special nature of the work that is so challenging to tease out.

Professionally and culturally, the order of the written word is safer and usually better respected than the chaos of the creative gesture, so the relationship between DMT and the verbal is understandably ambivalent. For example, the use of words, images, and drawing is owned by some practitioners whilst others are more tentative about admitting the role of the verbal in DMT. Penfield discusses the special qualities of movement and the body that are significantly different from linguistic and other representations.

If movement is treated only as a communication, only as a signifier or expression of something else, we forget that it also creates experience and meaning. Like the snake-skin, movement is more than a record of something else. We make an error either if we treat movement only as a map, an expression of a territory that it is the therapist's job to unearth, or if we treat it only as the territory, 'real experience', that is supposedly superior to words in its authenticity and directness.

Bateson again has a useful perspective, though he comments on non-verbal communication as a whole rather than movement alone:

> It seems that the discourse of non-verbal communication is precisely concerned with matters of relationship – love, hate, respect, fear, dependency, etc. – between self and vis-à-vis or between self and environment and that the nature of human society is such that

falsification of this discourse rapidly becomes pathogenic. From an adaptive point of view, it is therefore important that this discourse be carried on by techniques which are relatively unconscious and only imperfectly subject to voluntary control.

(Bateson 1973: 388)

Bateson draws attention to two main points. First, non-verbal communication is 'about' relationship, an intangible and invisible but real world of process and of connections between people and their world. This world may be ignored or distorted through verbal language, which tends, for example, to nominalize processes (thus 'love' and 'hate' are nouns and are discussed as objects; Bandler and Grinder (1975), building on the work of Bateson and of Noam Chomsky, describe a number of such properties of verbal language).

Second, it is important that such 'relationship communication' remains involuntary. Bateson points out, for example, that otherwise the appearance of conscious intent is given to every aspect of our behaviour. Non-verbal communication, and its degree of congruence with verbal communication, can be a useful guide to a person's sincerity, certainty, or internal conflicts; falsification of what is being 'said' through non-verbal communication may also create pathology, as in the 'double bind' theory of schizophrenia (Bateson 1973: 173–98).

This perspective by no means completes the task of articulating the special nature of movement and DMT. What it may help to do is make sense of the fundamental difference between the nature of DMT, at least beyond the behavioural or 'Learning I' level, and the world in which therapy is expected to operate as a technique with predictable, controllable results. It is not simply a question of favouring different languages that are alternative methods of accessing the same phenomena and which, therefore, are mutually substitutable and translatable; according to Bateson, 'our iconic communication serves functions totally different from those of language and, indeed, performs functions which verbal language is unsuited to perform' (1973: 388). DMT honours the integrity of non-verbal communication, and works directly with its world. Verbal language can negate and classify; movement cannot, except through deliberate gesture, and is a language of connection and possibility – the holistic nature of movement, such that several issues of relationship can be expressed simultaneously as a Gestalt, is referred to by Penfield, and Steiner refers to the possibility of synchronous expression in DMT versus diachronic expression in verbal therapy. Thus, the perspectives offered by non-verbal communication and verbal language are distinct, enabling complementary and sometimes contradictory understandings of experience.

Conclusion

The issue of DMT's identity has reflected the underlying theme of order and chaos through the efforts to clarify what DMT is and through the prospect that it cannot be defined easily. The snake-skin tells us that DMT is both young and old, both distinctive and related to the other fields, if not yet fully recognized. Its own medium and style have less need for language although the profession seems to desire articulation; however, the more explicit DMT becomes, the more its practitioners seem to sense it being forced into either standing apart from other therapies, thus shrinking its territory, or belonging to all of them, so having no separate identity. This could be a double bind, a situation in which DMT would lose whatever the outcome, but perhaps only if it is believed that DMT must be both explicit and certain, always choosing order over chaos. DMT may be learning to treat tensions between order and chaos, and between movement and words, as ironies rather than as obstacles; its domain not its bane.

THE THEORY AND PRACTICE OF DMT

Identity is an issue about DMT as a whole. This section explores issues of DMT's theory and practice, pursuing the basic theme of order and chaos in its approach to working with clients. There are, however, strong resonances of the issues of DMT's identity and being, demonstrating connections between different levels of meaning of the metaphorical snake-skin.

The five headings of this section are categories that seemed to capture the most prominent and significant issues of theory and practice. Between them they address all the themes listed in Table 12.1; they are present, I suspect, in every contributor's account and so may be fundamental to DMT. They lead as if on a spiral from the concept of 'synchrony', which is about external wholeness, similarity, and difference, through concepts of interaction, 'containers', and 'relationship', to 'meaning', which concerns the relationship of movement and language. The spiral returns to a theme of 'the energy of wholeness' in the final section, this time the inward wholeness and integration both of DMT clients and of DMT itself.

a) Synchrony

I was struck by the frequency with which 'synchrony' appears in the text. Although it is a key practical concept of DMT, I wonder about its significance in two other ways; the first is its identification with order (Table 12.1) and its implied relationship to chaos, and the second concerns the way DMT works with differences.

Some accounts in the book give instances of difference as something to be reduced. For example, Meekums talks of 'interactional synchrony as an indicator of empathy'. Stanton refers to the 'dampening down' of psychotic material; and Liebowitz connects synchrony and congruence. MacDonald talks of rhythm bringing order: 'because dance is rhythmic movement it is a wonderful tool to bring order into disordered lives.' Steiner links the asynchronous to fragmentation and depression and contrasts irregularity or lack of unity with flow, joy, and moving in synchrony.

Harmony can also mean conformity, the demand to be normal. Earlier, the risks of splitting were noted; it is also possible to deny difference, to seek a unity that collapses rather than transcends polarities. Stanton talks of a pressure for a group to 'synchronize, and for movements to become more standardized within the group', and reports in the case study a 'deviant' from the group who is referred to as asynchronous. She also refers to being a member of a group as a 'corrective emotional experience' that 'recapitulates the family grouping'.

Rhythm and synchrony seem strongly linked. Stockley refers to rhythm engendering group unity and belonging together with a sense of being an individual, and MacDonald talks of rhythm being used to maintain a sense of self to the exclusion of others. Although at first glance this may seem a contradiction of other references to synchrony and rhythm, the examples are connected by the use of rhythm to create order. MacDonald's example is of a client who used rhythm to establish a strong personal boundary; Steiner also refers to the power of group synchrony to function as a container of anxieties.

Synchrony seems to be treated more explicitly, more significantly, and perhaps more as an end in itself, where DMT is working on a more practical and concrete level. This contrasts with synchrony and asynchrony as a rhythm in the journey towards integration, where there is a higher-order concept corresponding to synchrony (wholeness or individuation) that goes well beyond the elimination of difference.

Synchrony and rhythm may therefore provide empathy, rapport, belonging, and safety; order that contrasts with the chaos of fragmentation and difference. Whilst the practical and theoretical subtleties of synchrony seem not to be articulated fully in this book, DMT is probably well equipped to understand order and chaos as a rhythm; perhaps there is a challenge to explore ways of using asynchrony and difference creatively, whatever the level of healing pursued.

b) Containers

The second theme concerns the nature, roles, and purposes of containers; a general issue of therapy, but with its own expression here. A tension in theory and practice is between, for example, structure and choreography (order) and freedom or improvisation within structure (chaos); these reflect themes of safety and risk, and of control. For example, some reported methods of working are much more structured than others; modifying behaviour through clear structures to reach specific outcomes seems safer and more contained than exploratory modes, parallel perhaps to the greater 'safety' of contained or bound movement and behaviour compared with free expression and deviance.

Container and contained, and the boundaries created between them, are reflected in many ways. The therapist herself can be seen as a container, bounding or directing the client's movement and exploration; the formal definition of DMT refers to the therapist's role of creating a holding environment. Sometimes this is obvious where there is explicit concern with control, whether pursuing an outcome of greater control for the client, as in the more behavioural level of working of Meekums (the client becomes 'more in control'), or in the sense of maintaining control of the DMT experience. Liebowitz talks of the therapist holding 'both physically and emotionally, the patient's body self together until such time as the psychotic can hold their own body self together through internalization of the maternal object'. She also refers to impulse control, self-regulation, and going out of control; and to the importance to a client of realizing the possibility of being 'in control'. Steiner talks of increasing control over life and of functioning independently, which recalls the reference above to the use of rhythm to establish independence.

Steiner, in contrast, also warns of the danger of the therapist over-containing or restricting, where 'those alienated from their bodies, who have no strong sense of self and are seldom able to focus on their centre as a source of energy and inspiration' . . . 'see the dance movement therapist as yet another person who is there to tell them what to do'.

Space is referred to as a container; Steiner especially talks of creating and safeguarding the therapeutic space, and of a safe climate for play and experiment. The group that inhabits the therapeutic space is talked of as a substitute mother – Payne refers to Bion on the mother as a container for difficult feelings. There is also frequent reference to the circle as a significant structure, encouraging both synchrony and safety, which derives from the work of Chace. Movement itself, as process, is therefore also a container. The preceding section described the way synchrony and rhythm could contain anxiety: 'a steady beat can help to provide a safe environment' (Steiner). Rituals are also referred to as providing a framework that both contains anxiety and clarifies boundaries.

Finally, the context within which DMT takes place can be a container. Meekums refers again to the 'holding environment'; Liebowitz discusses the 'holding experience' and the institution as a holding environment; Steiner talks of the clear boundaries and solid identity of the asylum; and Penfield refers to the therapeutic contract as a context for integration.

These different levels of container relate to Noack's discussion of the 'temenos', the protected precinct with three levels – outer space, body boundary, and self. Thus the institution, the therapeutic space, structure and rhythm, the client group and the therapist can all contain the client and the DMT process. In addition, the supervisor can be a container for the therapist (Penfield).

Improvisation, free expression, and spontaneity receive less direct attention but are in evidence in the case studies; I suspect they are more significant in practice than is suggested here. Penfield explicitly discusses improvisation as a working technique, and gives examples of clients' spontaneity. However, generally the emphasis seems to be more on containing and protection than on what happens within the container. Perhaps this reflects the need still for DMT practitioners to be acknowledged for their expertise at creating synchrony, harmony, and change, which might in turn allow them greater confidence to describe the more chaotic process and lower-key role of facilitation.

Containers in DMT therefore provide structure, creating both spaces in which things happen and boundaries that limit chaos. In practice, the choice is surely not between containment and improvisation, order or chaos alone; again, the challenge and the excitement of DMT seem to lie in the opportunities to move between and beyond this pair of opposites.

c) Relationship

Containers entail boundaries and some differentiation of what is inside from what is outside. Wilber points out that lines, such as the line formed by the shoreline and the sea, do not necessarily just separate one entity from another; they are the points at which differences touch and interact. Bateson (1973: 127) emphasizes the significance of seeing the world as connected and in relationship, not as relata – entities separated by boundaries – alone.

The accounts of DMT practice tell of much use of relationship in techniques, though most parallel similar techniques in counselling and therapy rather than being specific to movement work. Touching, perhaps the most basic form of such relating, is referred to specifically by Penfield and Steiner. Joining (Payne), empathy (the therapist taking on and experiencing a client's movement patterns), repetition, and echoing are described as forms of feedback, which can either damp down or amplify a client's movement. Liebowitz also refers to the therapist as mirror and feedback system; and mirroring, used consciously as a technique, is mentioned by Stanton and Penfield.

In a relationship-based model of therapist and client, difference and feedback – such as the echoing or countering of movement – develop the dance and its healing outcomes. The relationship is sometimes understood as a crucible in which the therapy takes place; hence transference and counter-transference, referred to by Liebowitz, Penfield, and others, are relational concepts. This would contrast with a model in which the therapist was felt to be a specialist, using techniques to produce effects in the client and being unaffected themselves.

The concept of relationship (central also to my approach to understanding patterns and problems in organizations) involves a different ordering or structuring of perceived reality, for example a boundary drawn around the therapist–client dyad rather than around each individual as an entity. Bateson's arguments about non-verbal communication being the principal medium for messages about relationship suggest that DMT is well suited to this theme. They also raise the question of whether, when DMT is ostensibly being used to develop a client's movement repertoire, it is more accurate to say that it is improving their relating repertoire.

d) Meaning

Earlier, the relationship of DMT with the verbal mode and with verbal psychotherapies was discussed in the context of identity. This section builds on the material about the distinctiveness of movement and non-verbal communication, but the interest is in the role of meaning and interpretation and in tensions between movement as ambiguity and chaos, and words as sense and order.

In any language or any symbol it is possible to find multiple levels of meaning. Liebowitz refers to the concrete and literal versus the metaphoric; Stockley talks of DMT embracing the sensory and the symbolic; and Stanton refers to levels described by Davis that recall the levels of meaning in the 'snake-skin': a) movement as illustration of an intrapsychic state, or communication to the therapist; b) movement as evidence (through rhythm and organization) of the developmental phase at which the patient has encountered difficulty; and c) movement as metaphor.

The use of movement for diagnosis and labelling, which may create a direct equivalence between the client's movement and categories such as 'schizophrenic', is firmly in the 'movement as evidence' category. Stanton says 'the difficulties of describing, classifying, and understanding movement pathology continue; recent approaches stress that motor and thinking abnormalities in mental illness may have a common pathogenic basis'. Liebowitz recognizes the possibility of the elucidation of defence mechanisms and of developmental stages from movement patterns.

Ramsden's Action Profiling is intentionally a more enabling, non-judgemental form of labelling that illustrates well the secret and complex nature of movement as a language. It differs, in its assumption that the basic patterns of movement and therefore the core being of the person do not change readily, from exploratory, symbolic approaches; but it also challenges the notion that changing a person's movement alone one may change the person.

Interpretation and labelling are not the only ways in which language is used to create order. Words can have a holding or containing function because they may reduce ambiguity, and verbalization can achieve a distancing and detachment that may be more difficult through movement. Stanton says: 'It is important not to quash the unconscious process, or interrupt the imagery and movement as it happens. However, it is important to assist the group in reflecting on their behaviour as it is happening, so as to prevent them merely releasing their feelings.' Steiner suggests that the therapist can voice the unspoken; this awareness means the client can be less at mercy of 'inner demons'.

Other material plays down the role of words and language. A strong theme in the book is of movement as 'evidence' of unconscious process, of emotion transformed into motion, and bodies and movement as symbols for feelings. Movement is something that yields imagery, something which can be explored to access the symbolic. 'Movement without words can also be analysed, and the communication contained within the quality of movement can be reflected back to the clients by therapist' (Stanton). Hesitation to verbalize is supported by Bateson's comments, cited above, about the dangers of translating kinesics or paralinguistic messages into words.

So far, the impression is that language and movement can coexist in DMT practice provided one of them is dominant. Are ambiguity and meaning, the non-verbal and the verbal, and the metaphorical and the literal, being treated yet as wholes? There is some evidence of DMT going beyond the poles of movement as either expression or material for interpretation. Steiner, for example, refers to the verbal and non-verbal leading to improvisation; and Noack talks of meaning being born from a creative cycle, an emergence of order from chaos that involves a very different emphasis from that of labelling.

Noack also refers to the numinous quality of movement, 'something sacred and bigger than the personalities involved and . . . frequently connected with the feeling-tone related to awe'. She explores the identity of Terpsichore as the offspring of Zeus, the light of consciousness, and Mnemosyne, who enables access to the past and the unconscious. This suggests again that language and movement may have complementary, creative roles rather than being competitors for the same task.

e) The energy of wholeness

The theme of integration in DMT theory and practice reconnects with that of DMT's own wholeness in this section. This reintroduces the issue of identity as well as completing the spiral from synchrony to wholeness, another meaning or version of synchrony at a different level.

The chapter's opening quotation about the snake and the trans-mutation of poisons towards integration has an inherent valuing of wholeness. DMT seems similar, on the evidence of this book: metaphors of circles, healing, synchrony, integration, wholeness, and transformation pervade it. There is also the alchemical and Jungian metaphor of the union of opposites (Noack).

Examples of themes of integration and wholeness in practice include Liebowitz's reference to 'unintegrated to integrated' and 'restoring parts to their rightful owner'. Penfield talks about integration through both organized movement and improvisation, giving the example of a 'movement overview'. Noack talks of integrated movement: 'the person governed only by time and social pressure is not in contact with the body spirit or the self'. The more DMT is concerned with the relationship between order and chaos the more it resembles other approaches like the Jungian. Rather than view the therapist as an agent, helping clients move from negative to positive or from chaos to order, where DMT is *about* the client's movement and wellness, DMT can be a dance itself, a spiral of order and chaos in which therapist and client join.

A metaphorical description of DMT process refers to 'excursion into unknown places' (Noack), a theme echoed for example in Kopp's (1974: 102) view of psychotherapy. An image of DMT that came to mind after reading several chapters of this book was of 'footsteps in the cellar'; as if it were living in an unknown place underneath a house and out of daylight, making faint noises that can be heard by the occupants, who are both curious and uneasy. This echoes the feel of DMT as something both ancient and unrecognized, as well as the sense in which the body and movement represent the shadow side of psychotherapy.

DMT is exploring unknown places now – overtly, articulation of its theory and practice and establishment of itself as a profession. Symbolically, I have speculated, the mother, and male energy, may represent the complement of DMT's existing identity. But I have suggested also that to seek out these aspects too avidly may be an error, tantamount to undervaluing the qualities of DMT's apparent existing strengths, its maiden and crone faces. My wish for more lightness and humour (which I have clearly not supplied myself) is unreasonable in the context of this book – they may exist in abundance, and more appropriately, within DMT practice – but is a concern about the evolution of DMT. Wilber comments that:

'progress' and unhappiness might well be flip sides of the same restless coin . . . the very urge to *progress* implies a discontent with the *present*. In blindly pursuing progress, our civilization has, in effect, institutionalized frustration.

(Wilber 1979: 20–1)

Can DMT, therefore, fully value its present identity, its qualities and balance of order and chaos, rather than institutionalize the frustration of denying its chaos to become articulated and structured? Can it honour and so contain the creative tension of difference both within its professional boundaries and in relation to other approaches, rather than mistake unity for wholeness? And can it apply to its own evolution the tolerance of ambiguity, the appreciation of multiple levels of meaning, and the perspective of relationship that exist within DMT practice?

CONCLUSION

This chapter has approached the book as a story through the metaphor of the snake-skin. It has tried to tease out patterns from the stories told by the contributors, looking at DMT both as a single entity and as a diverse collection of practices and philosophies. There have been parallels between DMT's content, its theory and practice, and its nature and development as an entity, different levels of meaning that are connected by the archetypal struggle of order and chaos.

As I finish the chapter I wonder what I have misunderstood, missed out, and overemphasized; perhaps this is a version of the desire to bring order out of chaos without the order being unnaturally and unreasonably imposed or the chaos being unappreciated. This partial perspective, one possible reading of the snake-skin, is therefore offered as a retelling and another layer of DMT's story.

REFERENCES

Bandler, R. and Grinder, J. (1975) *The Structure of Magic*, Palo Alto, CA: Science and Behaviour Books.
Bateson, G. (1973) *Steps to an Ecology of Mind*, London: Paladin.

——(1980) *Mind and Nature*, Glasgow: Fontana/Collins.
Bateson, G. and Bateson, M. (1979) *Angels Fear*, London: Rider.
Birdwhistell, R. (1970) *Kinesics and Communication*, University of Pennsylvania.
Hampden-Turner, C. (1981) *Maps of the Mind*, London: Mitchell Beazley.
James, T. and Woodsmall, W. (1988) *Time Line Therapy*, Cupertino: Meta Publications.
Kopp, S. (1974) *If You Meet the Buddha on the Road, Kill Him!*, London: Sheldon Press.
Sams, J. and Carson, D. (1988) *Medicine Cards*, Santa Fe: Bear & Company.
Starhawk (1982) *Dreaming The Dark*, Boston, MA: Beacon Press.
Tosey, P. C. (1986) 'Understanding change', Ph.D. thesis, University of Bath.
Wilber, K. (1979) *No Boundary*, Boulder, Colo.: Shambhala.
Woolger, J. and Woolger, R. (1990) *The Goddess Within*, London: Rider.

Afterword

Dance movement therapy began with a very few dedicated pioneers who worked in isolation until the late 1970s. Now it has a professional association and two validated training courses with qualified practitioners emerging each year. It has strong foundations with the richness of European dance and innovators such as Laban. The fertile soil surrounding approaches to group and individual therapy such as group-analytic, psychodynamic, and humanistic have provided the nourishment for DMT to grow. Our youth, in comparison with the other arts therapies, is a blessing in many ways for it allows us to be authentic and flexible as the flow of change necessitates new responses.

There may well be a different DMT practised a decade from now, with practitioners and students having access to more research, theoretical, and case study material, and a profession with registered members and which can be recognized with appropriate salaries and conditions of service.

This book is a start in the process of documenting UK theory and practice and represents a step out into a vacuum since currently there is no comparable publication. I hope it will be an initial movement towards greater sense-making and dissemination of our practice in DMT so that the efficacy of DMT continues to be explored, balanced with other approaches to research such as process-orientated enquiry. As our appreciation of the processes and outcomes of DMT evolves in this young/old profession it will change our practice. DMT is transforming in the UK and as such will be seen through different 'glasses' by practitioners and others.

Finally, DMT embodies both art and science and it is my hope that this has been reflected in this book.

Appendix

1 TRAINING

UK courses

There are two CNAA validated postgraduate training in dance movement therapy. The first course to be validated is located at *Hertfordshire College of Art and Design, 7 Hatfield Road, St Albans, Herts*, where there are also art and dramatherapy trainings at both postgraduate diploma and MA levels. The other course is located at the *Laban Centre, Laurie Grove, New Cross, London, SE14 6NW*. Entry is normally at postgraduate level, for those with degrees in dance, physical education, or the social sciences with a proven interest and training in a movement or dance form. Students are usually over 25 years of age with some understanding and experience of DMT and personal therapy. Experience or qualifications in one of the caring services is essential.

Other European courses

Holland

Dr H. Petzold,
Integrative Movement Therapy,
Faculty of Human Movement Sciences,
Vrije Universiteit, Room H 637, v.d. Boechorstraat 9,
1081 BT Amsterdam.

Hogeschool Nijmegen (Course Leader: Marlies Hoogma),
afd. Kreatievetherapie,
Postbus 9020,
6500 JK Nijmegen,
Holland.

Germany

The Fritz Perls Institute,
Haaner Str, 100,
4006 Erkrath,
Germany.

Deutsches Institut für Tanzetherapie,
Rilkestrasse, 103,
D-5300 Bonn 3,
Germany.

France

Institut Supérieur de Reéducation Psychomotrice,
37 bis rue Rouelle,
75015, Paris,
France.

Sweden

University of Stockholm,
Byvagen 40,
133 OO Saltsjobaden,
Sweden.

Italy

Art Therapy Italiana, (Headquarters)
450–45th Street,
Brooklyn,
New York 11220.

Other courses

USA

Antioch/New England Graduate School,
103 Roxbury Street,
Keene,
New Hampshire 03431.

Hahnemann University,
230 N Broad Street,
Philadelphia, PA 19102.

Hunter College,
425 E 25th Street,
New York 10010.

New York University,
35 W 4th Street,
Ed 675,
New York 10003.

Pratt Institute,
East Building,
200 Willoughby Avenue,
Brooklyn,
New York 11205.

UCLA,
405 Hilgard Avenue,
Los Angeles,
Calif. 90024.

2 ADDRESSES

The Association for Dance Movement Therapy,
c/o Arts Therapies Department,
Springfield Hospital,
Glenburnie Road,
Tooting Bec,
London SW17 7DJ.

Arts Therapies Research Committee,
Chair, Helen Payne,
1, The Wick,
High Street,
Kimpton,
Herts SG4 8SA.

Standing Committee for Arts Therapies Professions,
Chair: Vera Vaserhelyi,
c/o Bloomfield Clinic,
Guy's Hospital,
St Thomas St,
London SE1 9RT.

Committee for Arts Therapies in Education,
Chair, Angela Fenwick,
115 Habberly Road,
Kidderminster.

3 JOURNALS

The following journals are useful reading:

American Dance Therapy Journal,
Suite 230,
2000 Century Plaza,
Columbia, Maryland 21044, USA.

The Arts in Psychotherapy,
20 Ridgecrest East,
Scarsdale,
NY 10583, USA.

1974 SESAME
Drama and Movement in Therapy
(Wethered) 1 yr, full-time
Kingsway Princeton FE College

Now at Central School of Speech & Drama

1975–1985
Association of Dance Therapists
20 wk part-time course (now defunct)

1983–1985
Attenborough Report
(Committee of Inquiry into Arts and
Disability)
Arts Therapies document

1985 Laban Centre
imported MCAT training
Hahnemann University, USA

summer schools with course staff

1987 Foundation Course
Hertfordshire College of Art
and Design
(1 evening per wk × 10 wks)

1988 1 evening × 20 wks
1989–

plans for 30 wks

1989 Laban Centre
Postgraduate Diploma
MA (CNAA), 2–4 yrs
part-time

1976 Laban Certificate in
Movement and Dance with
reference to Special Education
(Mieir), 1 yr full-time

1981– Laban Certificate in Dance in
the Community, 1 yr full-time

Dr Joanna Harris visiting teacher
Summer School and Intensives
1979/80/81

Association for Dance Movement
Therapy inaugurated 1982

Summer schools 1982–1988
with leading Americans such as
Joanna Harris, Mara Capy, Marcia
Leventhal, for example

Roehampton Institute non-validated
2 yr part-time Marcia Leventhal
directing and teaching
1987–1989

Hertfordshire College of Art &
Design, St Albans
1987–present Summer and
International Easter Schools in DMT
with leading practitioners from UK,
USA and Europe

1988 Hertfordshire College of Art &
Design, 2 yr part-time or 1 yr full
time postgraduate Diploma (CNAA
validated)
1988–present

The development and flow of DMT training in Britain

Name index

Subject index